Macrobiotics in Motion

Macrobiotics in Motion

Yin & Yang in Moving Spirals

by Betsy Polatin

Japan Publications, Inc.

Published by JAPAN PUBLICATIONS, INC., Tokyo and New York

Distributors:
UNITED STATES: *Kodansha International/USA, Ltd., through Harper & Row, Publishers, Inc., 10 East 53rd Street, New York, New York 10022.* SOUTH AMERICA: *Harper & Row, Publishers, Inc., International Department.* CANADA: *Fitzhenry & Whiteside Ltd., 195 Allstate Parkway, Markham, Ontario, L3R 4T8.* MEXICO AND CENTRAL AMERICA: *HARLA S. A. de C. V., Apartado 30–546, Mexico 4, D. F.* BRITISH ISLES: *International Book Distributors Ltd., 66 Wood Lane End, Hemel Hempstead, Herts HP2 4RG.* EUROPEAN CONTINENT (except Germany): *PBD Proost & Brandt Distribution bv, Strijkviertel 63, 3454 PK de Meern, The Netherlands.* GERMANY: *PBV Proost & Brandt Verlagsauslieferung, Herzstrasse 1, 5000 Köln 40, Germany.* AUSTRALIA AND NEW ZEALAND: *Bookwise International, 1 Jeanes Street, Beverley, South Australia 5007.* THE FAR EAST AND JAPAN: *Japan Publications Trading Co., Ltd., 1-2-1, Sarugaku-cho, Chiyoda-ku, Tokyo 101.*

First edition: October 1987

ISBN 0–87040–687–6

Printed in U.S.A.

This book is dedicated to my father, Doctor Sydney Polatin,
whom I admire so much because he constantly cares
for the health and well-being of others,
and to my mother, Edna Polatin,
who devotes her life to the unity and well-being of her family;
today a lost art.

Foreword

Human motion is a part of the ceaseless movement of the universe. When human motion is in harmony with the movement of the universe, it is demonstrated by sublime beauty and supreme peace. When it is not in harmony, it creates chaos and confusion.

The movement of the universe and therefore every motion which arises on this planet, including human motion, is spiralic—expansion/contraction, yin/yang, male/female, heaven/earth, outward/inward, action/rest, are only a few examples. When humanity acts as a symbol of the universe with the spirit of peace and compassion, embracing every being and every phenomena, it realizes health, peace, and happiness, and directly serves physical, emotional, and spiritual development.

The author of this book, Betsy Polatin, is one of the rare persons realizing this motion. Her way of eating and expression come from the macrobiotic view. For nearly twenty years she has studied with me about life and its eternal cycle in harmony with the movement of the universe. My associates and I sincerely hope this book will be read by many people who, in turn, will gain not only the knowledge and teachings of motion, but also the spirit and insight of what life is.

March 16, 1987

MICHIO KUSHI
Brookline, Massachusetts

Acknowledgements

Thanks to all the teachers with whom I have had contact. And thanks to the people, environments and situations that I have encountered. Arthur Perry and Albert Pesso were my first influential dance teachers. After them I studied with many people in the United States and abroad. The next large influence (for eight years) came from Frances Cott, a movement educator with a truly remarkable understanding of ballet and body mechanics.

Thanks to Bo-In Lee, a Boston-based yoga teacher, who for five years taught me the value of human understanding, wisdom, and love. Gratitude to his wife Nam-ye Lee also.

Thanks to all my Alexander teachers, Tommy Thompson, Helen Jones, David Gorman, and others for making me aware of the moment of freedom between stimulus and response. And to many others for their books (especially F.M. Alexander and Frank Jones, in spirit). A special thanks to Tommy for seven years of allowing space for discovery and direction; for day-to-day training; for his consistency; and most of all for teaching me that I have the ability to "free in response to. . . ."

And great thanks go to Michio Kushi, who for the past twenty years has provided an unending depth of wisdom, patience, strength, naiveté and love; for his training in the way of life for physical, mental and spiritual growth and understanding, for past, present and future lives for myself and for all humanity. And to Aveline Kushi for teaching me to cook, the hidden art.

And largest thanks and gratitude to my family: to my ancestors and parents for allowing me my own direction; to my brothers; to Leon Djerahian; and to my two most devoted fans, Daria and Ruby, my daughters, who put up with a mother who does something in addition to being a mother.

And others who helped me in one way or another to get this book together: Carolyn Heidenry, Donna Cowan, Dora Polihroneau, the Lexington Waldorf School, Allen Bourque, Edward Esko, and Jean Crown. Special appreciation to Mr. Iwao Yoshizaki and Mr. Yoshiro Fujiwara, respectively president and New York representative of Japan Publications, Inc.

Credits

Thanks to:
Donna Ahrend, for word processing and for improving my English.
Satyam Anando, for editing advice and his worldly stories.

Photos

Thanks to:
Gus Kayafas and John Marcy of Palm Press for taking most of the sequence photos (unless indicated otherwise), and for all the multi-strobe prints.
Doc Edgerton at M.I.T., for the use of his equipment and studio.

Gay Bodick, for taking all the outdoor sequence photographs.

Nancy Hill-Joroff, for taking all the sequence photos of the children

May Baldwin, for the flower and vegetable photos in Chapter 3, Section 2, and Figure 3 in Chapter 2.

Johnny's Selected Seeds 1987 catalog, for Figure 7 vegetable photo in Chapter 3, Section 2 (great seeds from Albion, Maine 04910).

Museum of Fine Arts, for the photo of *Kuan Yin in Pose of Royal Ease*, Chapter 2 (used with permission).

Alain Ando Hirsch, for the cooking photo of Aveline Kushi.

Models in Chapter 5

Thanks to:

Stephen Hurley, Section 1

Anna Taylor Freeman, Section 6

Marilyn Arnold, Section 7

Austin Lyons, Section 9

Leigh Freeman, Section 13

Daria Djerahian, Section 14A-1, sitting

Aladdine Joroff, Section 14A-1, lying down

Ruby Djerahian, Section 13A-1, in black pants

Jaimee Joroff, Section 13A-1, in overalls

Artwork

Thanks to:

David Gorman, for permission to reprint or adapt illustrations in Chapter 1 (see notes) from *The Body Moveable*.

Christian Gautier, for his illustrations, Chapter 1, Illustration 42; Chapter 5, Illustration 2.

Jane Mitcheson, for her drawing, Chapter 3, Illustration 2.

Melissa Sweet, for her professional advice.

[Note: Fig.=photographs; Illus.=drawing]

Contents

14

Introduction

"Truth is a pathless land. Man cannot come to it through any organization, through any creed, through any dogma, priest or ritual, not through any philosophic knowledge or psychological technique. He has to find it through the mirror of relationship, through the understanding of the contents of his own mind, through observation and not through intellectual analysis or introspective dissection."
—Krishnamurti

We all search for a formula to attain perfect health. Unfortunately, it does not exist. But there are principles to keep in mind: the whole, complementary opposites (motion–stillness), and spirals. There is also the given development, design and function of nature and the human body, manifest through movement.

The Taoist sage, Chuang Tzu, when still a disciple, was taken to a bridge over a fast-flowing river. He was told to stand on that bridge and stare at the water until it stopped and he moved.

Life is moving. Be it fast or slow, visible or invisible, small or grand, endless motion exists, moving at infinite and infinitesimal speed in all directions. We understand this movement through our bodies. The freer and more flowing we are in those bodies, the freer we will be in our lives to experience variety and delight in simple activities.

There are many paths that one may choose to approach this freedom. Some are more mechanical, some more intellectual, and some reflexive. One may suit your needs today, another five years from now. One may get rid of physical pain, another may lead to a fuller understanding of your life choices and the way you think about yourself. You may choose to suit your needs.

There are no set rules. Life is a spiral, and depending upon where you are, it determines your point of view. If I am "A" I see one way, and if I become "B" I see another way. (See Illus. 1.) For instance, if you look at a log straight on, it is round

Illus. 1

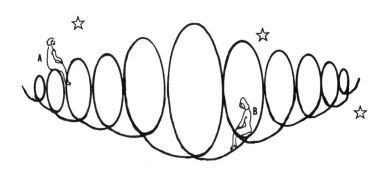

Fig. 1 **Fig. 2**

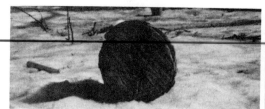 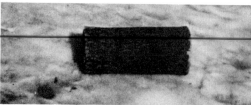

(Fig. 1), if you look at it sideways (Fig. 2), it is long and narrow. But it is the same log so both views are "correct" depending upon your vantage point.

We need to develop an overview to see the whole—the mental, the physical and the spiritual, which are already one; we must learn to be the whole that already exists.

Primitive men, our ancestors, grew or hunted their food, built their homes and took responsibility for their lives. Their daily lives naturally included appropriate diet, exercise and resting time. This resulted in a wholeness that developed their bodies and minds toward survival, or they perished. They followed the natural order.

Modern life is partial. The dizzying array of paces and directions are fragments of the whole, but we grab them as if they are the whole picture. For example, the current body-building craze is a perfect reflection of this obsession—one exercise for this muscle, another one for that one. We are unconsciously separating ourselves from the whole, leading to endless dissatisfaction. This dissatisfaction keeps us in constant motion toward something outside of ourselves. We are always searching, but for what we don't know.

We must learn to stop, listen and observe. We must consciously relearn how the body structure is designed to move in harmony with the universal wholeness and what foods best sustain the relationship.

"No pain, no gain" is the banner of the body builders. This book presents a gentler approach toward you and your body. Excess tension and pain restrict your movement and take you farther from your path of truth. Gautama Buddha often said, "Easy is right."

The book may seem to have sections that conflict in principle, but they are only different steps along the spiral of learning appropriate foods and movement. Those steps we may call the dance of life. For instance, in one section I explain in length that breathing is a reflex and we should only stop doing what we are doing and allow the breath to come in and out, without the *self* controlling it. Yet in another I give specific techniques for breathing in and out, and to different parts of the body.

I have done this only because individuals are at different stages of development. Some need more mechanical guidance (how to do, for instance), and some need intellectual explanations (this muscle does this, etc.). Some need to do, others can allow. Your choice is your dance.

Imperfections and inconsistencies exist. They are the complementary opposites that are part of the spiral and part of this book. Perfection needs imperfection to exist. They are two sides of the same thought process. They create what I call "spiralic thinking." This mode of thinking allows spiral movement. This is in contrast to linear thinking and movement which injure the body and mind. Exercises that only flex and extend leave out the spiral design of the muscle. They also chain the mind to a black *or* white point of view. With this they miss the union, the breathing space where the complementaries—opposites like balance and imbalance, salty and sweet—meet.

These ideas do not represent the whole of the macrobiotic community nor the whole of the Alexander community, but they are the author's synthesis and lifelong observations. These observations denote no value judgment, just observations and correlations. There is no good or bad implied. There is nothing to "get," only something to "allow."

My personal view is that we are healthier the more we can consciously leave ourselves alone, stop pulling and adjusting our muscles, and let the forces of heaven and earth, brought out by the reflexes, relay our movements. Since that is difficult for many people, the sequences and explanations given provide steps to reach this.

It is my hope that this book will provide insight, direction and clarity for our existence, and flexibility to solve our problems. I intend no dogma or set creed, just tools to be used and when no longer needed, abandoned.

July, 1984

1. Nature and the Human Body

"Man grows and moves spirally."
—Raymond Dart[1]

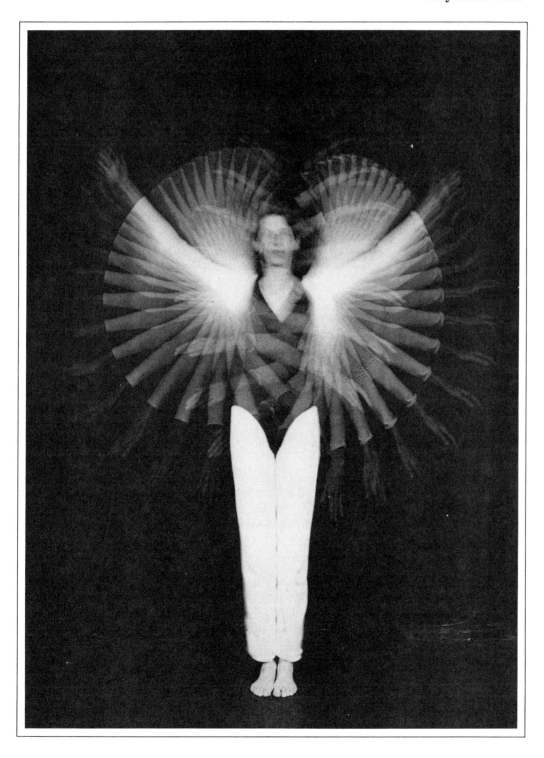

1. Spirals of the Uniuverse

Motion exists because of polarity between high-pressure–low-pressure systems, positive–negative flow, and expansion–contraction. As sensing, thinking and acting human beings we see and feel this motion from the total body: physical, mental, emotional, and spiritual. We understand this movement through the stage of physicalization that we call the body.

We have physical form because we eat physical food, mainly from the vegetable kingdom. The vegetable or plant kingdom is made up of various elements. The elements are made up of pre-atomic particles (electrons, neutrons, etc.). The pre-atomic particles are made up of vibration and energy. Energy is made up of polarization (two forces). Polarization is made from wholeness or infinity. The journey is a dance all along the way from one infinity to our physicalized being (1–7) (Illus. 1).

Illus. 1

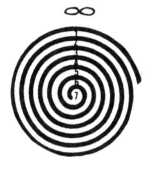

1 God, One Infinity
2 Polarization
3 World of Vibration
4 Preatomic Particles
5 World of Elements
6 Vegetable Kingdom
7 Animal Kingdom

The infinite is wholeness and absolute, including everything and anything with no beginning and no end. From here two poles arrise. This is the beginning of all relative phenomena and motion.

Some ancient philosophies called the poles yin and yang. To most modern people these terms are a bit difficult because you cannot see, feel or do yin or yang. They are only tendencies, directions, or states for degrees of comparison of antagonistic

Examples of Yin and Yang[2]

	Yin Centrifugal Force	Yang Centripetal Force
Tendency	Expansion	Contraction
Function	Separation	Gathering
Movement	Inactive or slower	Active or faster
Direction	Ascent or vertical	Descent or horizontal
Position	Outward-periphery	Inward-central
Weight	Lighter	Heavier
Temperature	Colder	Hotter
Humidity	More wet	More dry
Biological	More vegetable quality	More animal quality

and complementary phenomena. These poles govern the large order that pervades our universe and the principles of eternal change. This understanding is not a technique, but is the core which endlessly creates every technique.

George Ohsawa, teacher and philosopher, healer and active, contemporary worldly seeker of justice and the truth, put together seven universal principles of the infinite universe. He followed those with twelve laws of change of the infinite universe.

Seven Principles of the Order of the Universe

1. Everything is a differentiation of One Infinity.
2. Everything changes.
3. All antagonisms are complementary.
4. There is nothing identical.
5. What has a front has a back.
6. The bigger the front, the bigger the back.
7. What has a beginning has an end.

Twelve Theorems of the Unifying Principle

1. One infinity manifests itself into complementary and antagonistic tendencies, Yin and Yang, in its endless change.
2. Yin and Yang are manifested continuously from the eternal movement of one infinite universe.
3. Yin represents centrifugality, Yang represents centripetality. Yin and Yang together produce energy and all phenomena.
4. Yin attracts Yang. Yang attracts Yin.
5. Yin repels Yin. Yang repels Yang.
6. Yin and Yang combined in varying proportions produce different phenomena. The attraction and repulsion among phenomena is proportional to the difference of the Yin and Yang forces.
7. All phenomena are ephemeral, constantly changing their constitution of Yin Yang forces; Yin changes into Yang, Yang changes into Yin.
8. Nothing is solely Yin or solely Yang. Everything is composed of both tendencies in varying degrees.
9. There is nothing neutral. Either Yin or Yang is in excess in every occurrence.
10. Large Yin attracts small Yin. Large Yang attracts small Yang.
11. Extreme Yin produces Yang, and extreme Yang produces Yin.
12. All physical manifestations are Yang at the center, and Yin at the surface.

These may sound overwhelming on first reading, but intuitively we know and can understand their truth, for we continuously see manifestations of them in our daily lives. As much as we might like to, we cannot deny them, for all phenomena exist in accordance with them and are changing according to them. Nature makes balance immediately. When the room is hot, we open the window and cool air comes in.

Nothing can continue to expand forever, it would explode eventually. Day changes to night, youth changes to old age, and before any leap upward there is a bend of the knees. Happy moments melt into moments of despair and back again to happy, as is readily observable in the behavior of children. Both sides are automatically there, and there is movement between the two.

"What has a front has a back." To outsiders, life for a celebrity seems glamorous, but we also know that many difficulties, injuries, fears, and pains exist in such a life. In Cary Grant's heyday, everybody wanted to be like him. When responding to this, Grant said, "I also want to be like Cary Grant." Even in our human bodies, the front has a charming face and sensual sexual organs, while the back has a head of hair and the exit for all waste products.

With this perspective we know that all manifestations in this universe can be observed and understood as either yin or yang in relationship to each other. Knowing these laws we can live with the justice of the kingdom of heaven. Using them we can change sickness to health. Living them we can change chaos to order. To deny or ignore them brings unhappiness and futility. Through this we can understand that there is no injustice in life or nature, just a striving to restore balance and to continue.

The interaction between these two poles creates a twist or spiral, which becomes the pattern of motion for all manifestations. At every junction where two forces meet, a spiral is formed. Spiralic energy currents are flowing everywhere. This spiral, a combination of what we call a spiral, a sphere, and a circle, is the universal motion. The earth is rotating within itself and revolving around the sun. The whole Milky Way galaxy is a spiral, spiraling around another spiraling galaxy, and so forth. If our health is tuned, we can catch the spiral wave and glide with no effort.

In ancient times men who lived in the mountains were said to fly. This phenomena is similar to a high jump or great leap or a child playing—riding the spirals of the universe.

The spiral moves within the body. Oxygen comes in and carbon dioxide goes out, the heart beats and blood flows. The body moves in space on these arcs, from batting an eyelash to grand movements of the limbs and torso. If continued, every body movement turns into a spiral. With this we can make shapes in space that are graceful or grotesque, skillful or clumsy. We can stamp in anger, curve in love, retreat in fear, and advance in confidence. Teachers, cowboys, actors, cooks, businessmen, pilots, drunks, and athletes all spiral their bodies and the space around themselves in different ways. Yet the spiralic structure of the human body is the same in all of us.

Spirals are seen in everything in nature: water down the drain, a seashell, a spider web, fingerprints, a DNA molecule, or rings on a tree. The list goes on, the spiralic formation of the universe is displayed in every creation of nature. Only where man has imposed his will on nature, such as in manufacturing synthetic or chemically made products, is the spiral lost.

A.   Spirals in the Body

Basic spiral formation:
All organic growth is created by two sets of spirals, which move in opposite directions, one clockwise and one counterclockwise. To see this, first look at a series of concentric circles on a logarithmic scale with straight lines radiating from the center

Illus. 2

Illus. 3

Illus. 4

Illus. 5

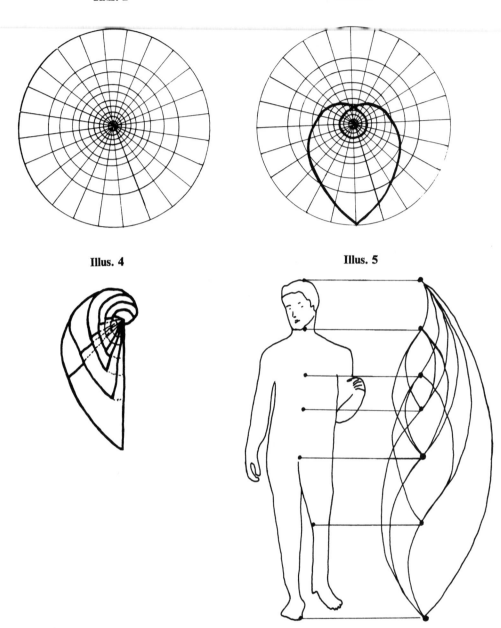

(Illus. 2). Connecting meeting points of these two sets of lines we see growth of the spirals that is logarithmic and equiangular (Illus. 3). In Illustration 4 we isolate one spiral.

By connecting different points, these basic spirals can create triangles, rectangles, squares, and other forms with these harmonious angles and proportions. These patterns and angles can be seen in flowers, plants, animals, and humans (Illus. 5).[3]

Illustration 6 shows the cross section of the core of an *axoneme* (minute elements in living cell structure), enlarged 90,000 diameters. The double spiral arrangement is clear.[4]

Illus. 6   **Illus. 7**

Illus. 8

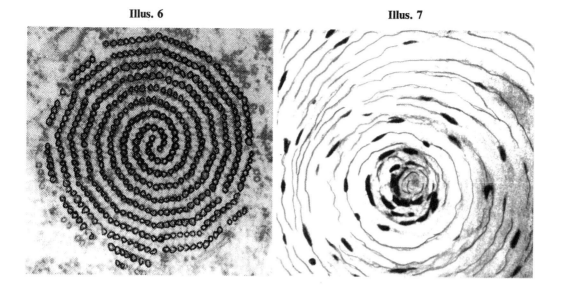

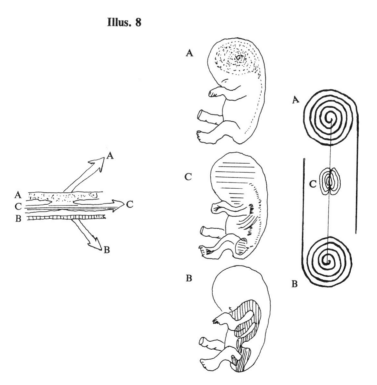

Illustration 7 is a drawing of an enlarged corpuscle of a sensory receptor. The dark dots in the bands are nuclei in the cells.[5]

Three embryonic germ layers[6] (Illus. 8):

nervous system—*ectoderm*—A

circulatory including

urinary system—*mesoderm*—C

digestive system (glands)—*endoderm*—B

Our three basic systems have a spiralic formation.

In the body there are seven spiralic meeting places called *chakras*, or energy centers (Illus. 9):

1. crown—top head
2. third eye—forehead
3. throat
4. heart
5. solar plexus
6. *tanden*—sacral
7. base—sexual organ

On every human head we see one or sometimes two head spirals (Fig. 1):

Illus. 9

Fig. 1

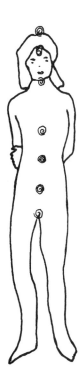

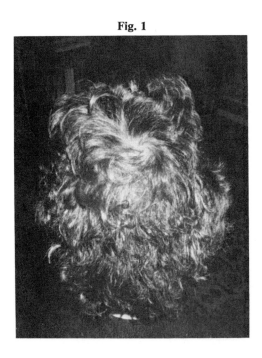

The seven energy centers, or chakras, form a vertical channel for the flow of electro-magnetic energy between heaven and earth.

B. Spirals in Bone Structure

Spiral of the arm (Fig. 2 and Illus. 10):
1. root—collar bone and shoulder blade
2. upper arm
3. forearm
4. palm
5. bottom finger joint
6. middle finger joint
7. top finger joint

Another way to see this is the 1-2-3-4-5 arrangement of the bones in arms and legs (Illus. 11):
1. upper arm
2. forearm

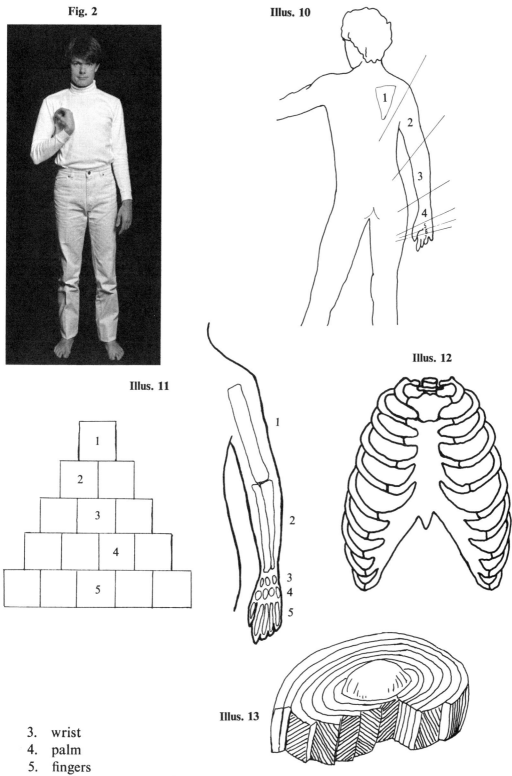

Fig. 2

Illus. 10

Illus. 11

Illus. 12

Illus. 13

3. wrist
4. palm
5. fingers

Spirals can also be seen in the rib cage and in the spine. It is not so easy to see in the bony part (the vertebrae). But it is very clearly seen if we examine an intervertebral disc, the rubber-like plate between the vertebrae (Illus. 12 and 13).[7]

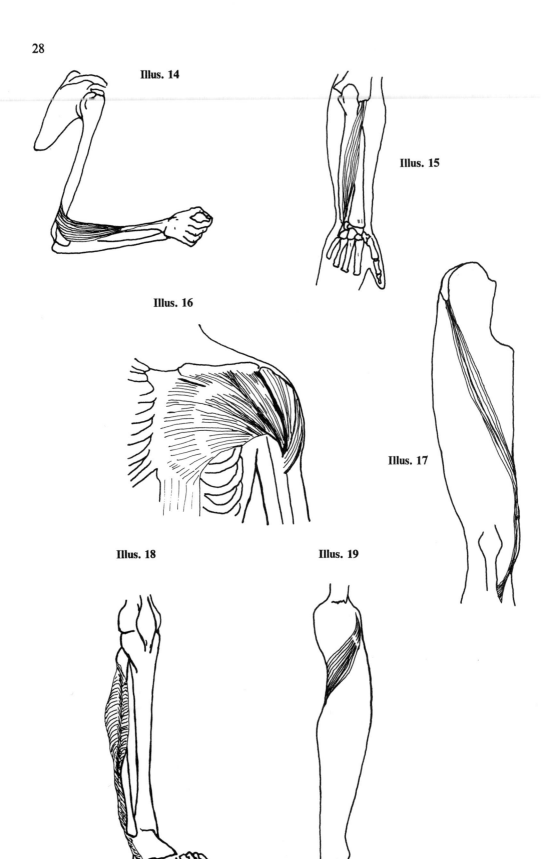

Illus. 14

Illus. 15

Illus. 16

Illus. 17

Illus. 18

Illus. 19

C.   Spirals in the Muscles[8]

Spiral muscles of the arm:
Illustration 14 is brachio radialis.
Illustration 15 is extensor carpi ulinaris.
Illustration 16 is a front view of the pectoralis major, the deltoid, and the biceps.
Spiral muscles of the leg:
Illustration 17 is a front view of the sartorius.
Illustration 18 is the peroneus longus.
Illustration 19 is a back view of the popliteus.
Spiral muscles of the back (Illus. 20):
A is the trapezius.
B is the latissimus dorsi.
C is the gluteus maximus.
Spiral muscles of the front:
1.   The abdomen:
Illustration 21 is the right side view of the external oblique.
Illustration 22 is the right side view of the internal oblique.

Illus. 20

Illus. 21

Illus. 22

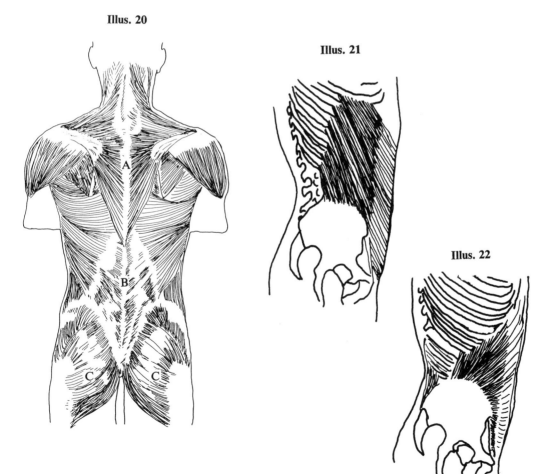

30

Illus. 23

Illus. 24

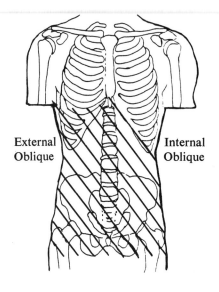

External Oblique   Internal Oblique

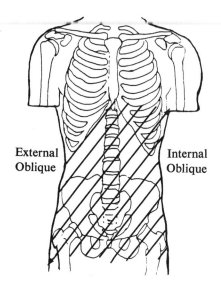

External Oblique   Internal Oblique

Illus. 25

Illus. 26

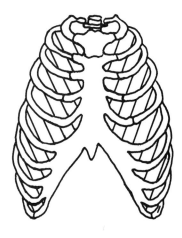

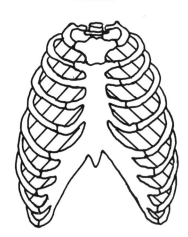

Illus. 27

Illus. 28

External Intercostals   Internal Intercostals

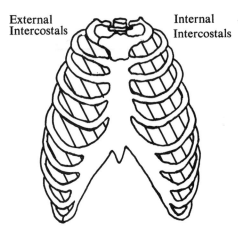

Internal Intercostals   External Intercostals

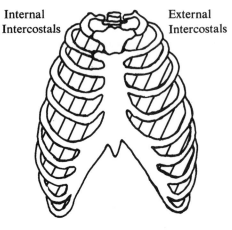

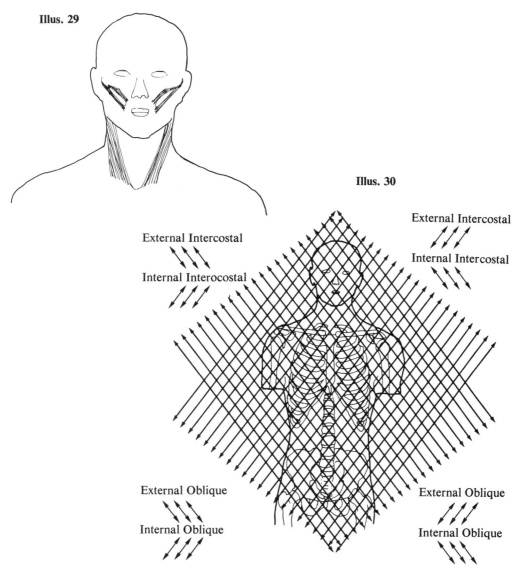

Illus. 29

Illus. 30

External Intercostal

External Intercostal

Internal Intercostal

Internal Interocostal

Internal Interocostal

External Oblique

External Oblique

Internal Oblique

Internal Oblique

Illustration 23. The right side external oblique and left side internal oblique form a diagonal.

Illustration 24. The left side external oblique and right side internal oblique form a diagonal.

2. The chest:

Illustration 25 is the external intercostals.

Illustration 26 is the internal intercostals.

Illustration 27. The right external intercostal and left internal intercostal form a diagonal.

Illustration 28. The left external intercostal and right internal intercostal form a diagonal.

Spiral muscles of the neck:

Illustration 29 is the sternocleidomastoid on the bottom and the zygomaticus major and minor on the top.

Together the flow lines look like this (Illus. 30):

Illus. 31   **Illus. 32**   **Illus. 33**

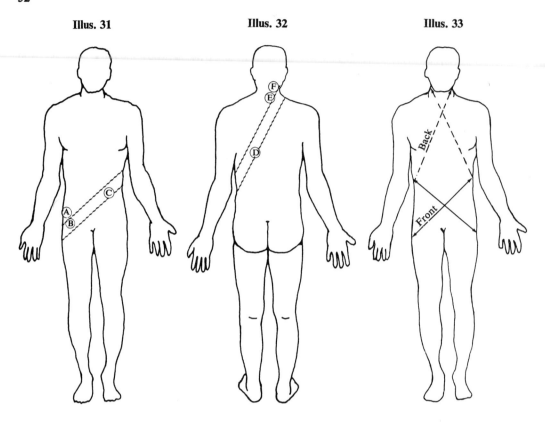

Torso spiral patterns:

Torso spirals—We can see large spiralic muscle groups if we examine the way individual muscles work together. One side only is shown for clarity.

Front—from bottom right side to top right side:

A. right hipbone iliac crest
B. to internal obliques
C. to external obliques, to
D. external intercostals underblade
E. splenius to
F. right mastoid process

Illustration 31 shows A, B and C. Illustration 32 shows D, E and F. Illustration 33 shows all together.

Back from top left side to bottom left side:

A. left mastoid process
B. front sterno mastoid
C. internal intercostals
D. latissimus dorsi
E. gluteus maximus
F. to left hip bone

Illustration 34 shows A, D, E and F.
Illustration 35 shows B and C.
Illustration 36 shows them together.

Illus. 34   Illus. 35   Illus. 36

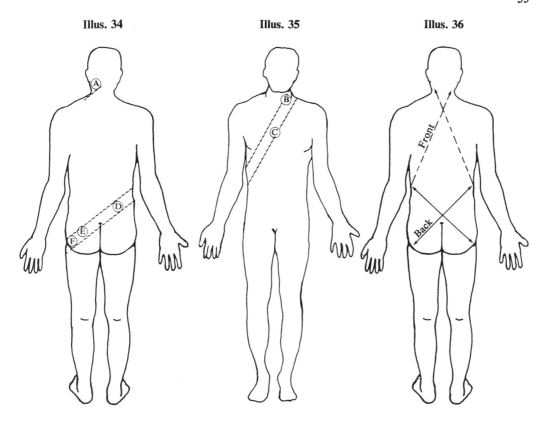

These two large spiral patterns (Illus. 33 and 36) put together form a simple version of what is called the double helix spiral pattern. These patterns can be seen evolving from the sinuous body motion in fish: while one side expands, the other contracts. This produces locomotion. The same may be said for bilateral human beings. As you step on one leg to walk, one side shortens while the other lengthens. Then you step on the other foot and they reverse. This spiralic pattern also governs our movement bias—right handed or left handed. These spirals are affected by breathing, locomotion and organ function.

D.   The Work of Raymond Dart

Professor Raymond Dart, the distinguished anthropologist, Emeritus Professor of Anatomy and Dean Emeritus of the Medical Faculty at the University of Witwatersrand, and present Chairman at "The Institute of Man" in Philadelphia, wrote an article entitled "Voluntary musculature in the human body: the double spiral arrangement."[9] The article begins:

> I recall an elderly otologist named Miller, 30 years ago in New York City demonstrating, by means of examples ranging from the spiral nebulae to the human cochlea and from the propagation of sound to the propulsion of solid bodies, that all things move spirally and that all growth is helical.

Dart continues to explain how spiral development occurs. In the evolution of voluntary musculature the first division is bilateral arrangement of *somites* (block-like cellular groupings) in which alternating contractions of the entire musculature on both sides produce lateral bending (Illus. 37). This is evident as early as the second week after conception.

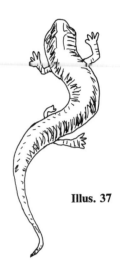

Illus. 37

Davenport Hooker discovered that such lateral (side to side) bending is the first reflex movement to appear in the human fetus. It appears after the eighth week only in response to stimulation of the upper lip and the alae of the nose. It is important because:

1)   it is the oldest and functionally most important reflex pattern involving the head and body segments, and

2)   it is the movement which brings the creature in contact with its food supply.

The second division of the segmented bilateral musculature is the front and back splitting of each segment into an extensor (those behind) and a flexor (those in front of the center of our vertebrae) half on each side of the body. This was accompanied by division of the spinal nerves into front and back.

Ancestrally there are only two sorts of striped muscular responses. Flexion and extension are the only alternative movements that any muscle can perform. So all our muscles were and still are either extensors or flexors. Rotational movement is the result of interaction between them.

These developments enabled the flexor halves of the somites on both sides of the body to contract or relax, separately or as a whole, independently from and antagonistically to the relaxing or contracting extensor halves of the somites. This is evident in the human embryo at five weeks of life. Simply put, as soon as it is possible to maintain one end of the body in a state of flexion or contraction, while the other end is in a state of tonic extension or lengthening, a postural twist results between the two ends. Developmentally speaking, most muscles are formed this way and most movement is based on these twists.

Further development and layering of these muscles display Dart's view of the double spiralic arrangement which is of fundamental importance to the upright body of a human being. Only one side of the double spiral is shown.

Illustration 38 is a side view.

Illustration 39 is a front view.

Illustration 40 is a back view.

The arrangement of the trunk musculature in the form of interwoven double spiral sheets characterizes the voluntary musculature of the trunk. Thus, the head and vertebrae suspend the body by means of these two spiral sheets of muscle encircling the trunk. In Dart's words,

> The majority of people—as a result of their single-handedness and their fixed and frequently sedentary occupations, to say nothing of their food and clothing—suffer from mild, moderate and even serious grades of permanent postural twist, although the condition has not been recognized by themselves or by their medical advisors.[10]

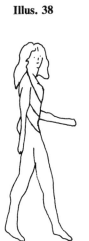

Illus. 38

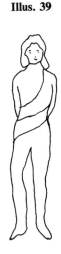

Illus. 39

Illus. 40

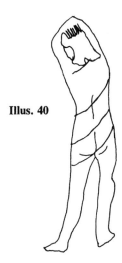

Dart used the double spiral arrangement to greatly improve health conditions in his own family. Conditions ranging from exhaustion to spastic movement, to a child's nightmares. Dart's work as an acclaimed anatomist and scientist coincides with the natural spiralic order of the universe—nature and science as one.

2. Yin and Yang of Becoming Human[11]

Between yin and yang is a spiral. In biological development, the yin or centrifugal force became the vegetable kingdom and yang or centripetal force became the animal kingdom. Thus, any movement observed in plants, such as trees swaying in the wind, is more yin or passive. On the other hand, movements from the animal world, like a tiger pouncing on its prey, are more yang or active. The yang creatures ate yin plants or animals that were more yin than themselves. Within the evolution of the plant and animal kingdoms we see yin and yang rolling in and out, paving the way. At the extreme, yin will change to yang and vice versa. (See Illus. 41.)

We begin our observation with an amorphous structure that saw food and made a temporary mouth, and then a temporary stomach, and finally an exit for waste. This sea invertebrate ate (and still eats) sea moss. At this stage we begin to see two major instincts that have continued throughout evolution in all animals, including human beings:

1) the instinct to expand (yin), to move into the world, and
2) the instinct to contract (yang) or stabilize, or to find security at home.

We have a built-in equilibrium between these two. We like to feel secure and comfortable yet we seek freedom and adventure.

Our creature then began to differentiate (yin), creating systems for specific jobs: 1) a digestive tube, a one-directional system, constructed so food could enter, digest, and exit as waste at the other end (front and back); 2) a circulatory system to spread

36

Illus. 41

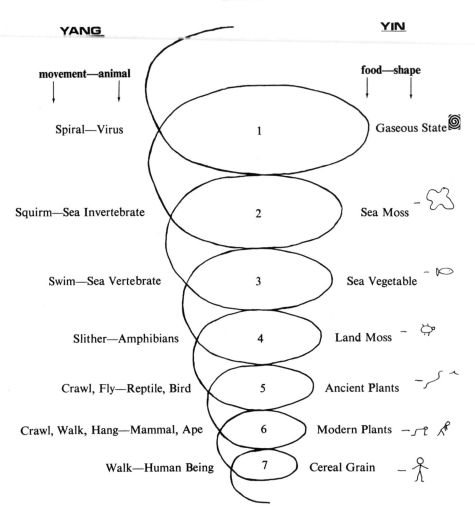

YANG

YIN

movement—animal

food—shape

Spiral—Virus	1	Gaseous State
Squirm—Sea Invertebrate	2	Sea Moss
Swim—Sea Vertebrate	3	Sea Vegetable
Slither—Amphibians	4	Land Moss
Crawl, Fly—Reptile, Bird	5	Ancient Plants
Crawl, Walk, Hang—Mammal, Ape	6	Modern Plants
Walk—Human Being	7	Cereal Grain

all this food and nourishment out (spirals); and 3) a nervous system or something to coordinate it all (up and down).

Now because of these differentiations he needed a new shape or form (yang) to keep things in place. Connective tissue kept him from coming apart, bones maintained the shape and muscles moved the creature.

Our creature until this point was more or less radial, like a starfish. But the sea vertebrate then became bilateral because of 1) the lengthening of the vertebral column (yin) and 2) segmented musculature (yang) for locomotion like a fish.

The bones were then used for walls of the container (yin—passive) and for leverage to help muscles in movement (yang—active). David Gorman, a functional anatomy and Alexander teacher, calls the spine a distortion joint. This means that any move-ment changes the whole thing, and when the movement is finished it always wants to return to its original shape.

Up to this point there are no flexible joints; then, the first to come along . . . the jaw. The first freely movable joint was a thickening and condensing of the front gill, enabling our sea creature to get higher-quality food more actively. The sea vertebrate then ate sea vegetables and smaller kinds of animals.

This creature had two pairs of fins that will be limbs: 1) arms (more yin, upper and freer), and 2) legs (more yang, lower and supportive). Along with these fins came more developed air sacs (later lungs), enabling him to swim more toward the surface (more yin).

Our creature then found himself on land—an amphibian (more yang)—and began to find a way to support himself. For this the fins gradually became the 1-2-3-4-5 bone arrangement. The spine curved to prevent the lungs and digestive organs from being squashed. The amphibian eats land moss and some insects. As breathing (lungs) moved down, a clearer neck appeared, so we had a head that could move separately from the body (yin and yang). As the organs developed, the torso had more of a container job (yin) and less locomotion, while the limbs took over locomotion (yang).

Next came reptiles and birds (more yin). They took the limbs from the sides of the body, and brought them down under the body and closer together. This developed biped motion, yin and yang in harmony. Evolution also eventually produced warm blood, a partial palate to separate eating and breathing, and a sealed egg so animals were not tied to the water. Reptiles primarily eat ancient plants like ferns, as well as some other animals.

The mammals (more yang) took some back muscles, created the diaphragm, and made a smaller and more efficient breathing system. This made room for internal birth (yang), making them more mobile: they didn't have to stay in one place for the egg to develop. This development demanded a more organized central nervous system which also allowed the mammals freedom to grow after birth. In contrast, reptiles are completely programmed from birth.

Then came the primates who lived in the trees (more yin). The sense-dominance changed at this time from smell to sight (yin). The cerebral front brain (yin) was developed as primates used their arms more for hanging and swinging from the trees and they refined their hand grasping. The upper body (yin) developed because of the rotation needed in the arm for swinging from trees. The apes eat modern plants like fruits.

Then we find ourselves back on the ground as humans (more yang). The over-developed upper body (ribs) spread back around the spine. Because of ground use, the legs and pelvis get longer and more balanced in the upright instability. And the extensor muscles down the back and in back of the lower leg develop more to keep us upright. The head is out of balance and consequently must be brought back to balance. We have a greatly developed brain to receive distant vibrations or to control the world around us. The foods for human beings are primarily cooked cereal grains and secondarily, because of our freedom, anything we choose.

I think the next stage of evolution, which has already happened for some people and is happening for others, is recognizing the spiritual order (more yin). Members of this species of human beings are consciously trying to understand the order of the universe and themselves and harmonize the relationship. They live a creative, joyful and non-competitive life.

Most accepted theories on evolution concentrate on heredity and environment but overlook what I consider an equally essential factor: food. Food is a means of evolution. By changing our food we change ourselves. For example, if an animal moves to a warmer climate, he begins to eat the vegetation around him. He begins to change and his offspring are correspondingly different. Over the generations a new species evolves, well suited to the warmer weather. This can be seen with people also. Black people living in Africa are baked by the hot sun and eat tropical yin foods. When they move to America, a colder climate with more yang foods, their color becomes less dark over the centuries.

I further suggest that evolution is, has been and will continue to be a harmonizing between the species—his food and environment—and not, as has been emphasized, a fight to the finish in which only the fittest survive.

3. Yin and Yang of Being Human

Now we have arrived at human form—two eyes, two nostrils, one mouth, two arms, two legs, and so on. The similarities are great but the differences are bigger. No two people are alike, perhaps a parallel to the vastness of the universe of which we are part. Illustration 42 is a drawing from *Life* nature books, showing the resemblance between the universal form and human form.

Humans are categorized in so many ways according to birth (time and place), body structure, temperament, movement preference, elements, colors, sense dominance, and even planetary influence. Most classifications have between two and twelve categories. As part of this whole we contain shades of all characteristics, but one will dominate. Traits came to have associations with different parts of the body, thus producing different movement habits. The following classifications are intended to allow students to see themselves in many ways and to choose to develop an area that may need attention. For example, you might read Rudolph Steiner's classifications and term yourself a "melancholic." When you become aware of those tendencies, you may choose to think about or do the recommended sequences or diet and perhaps you will gradually experience more wholeness and become less attached to the melancholic aspect of yourself. By changing your motion you may change your emotion. Some dietary and movement recommendations are presented to correlate with the following chapters. Check the bibliography for book titles to learn more about these subjects, as only the barest facts are presented in this context.

Classification I

On hearing of the way, the best of men
Will earnestly explore its length.
The mediocre person learns of it
And takes it up and sets it down.
But vulgar people, when they hear the news,
Will laugh out loud, and if they did not laugh,
It would not be the way.[12]

—Lao-tzu

Illus. 42

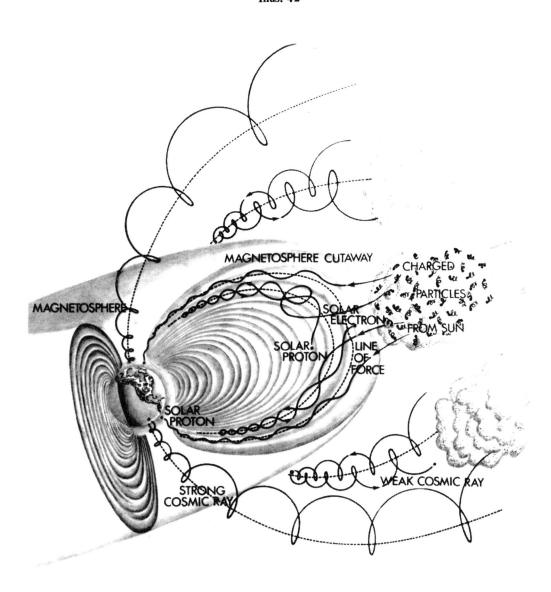

The One, the Infinite, God, Supreme Being, Allah, Jaweh. Every culture has
a symbol for the oneness. It is the uniqueness of each individual and the sameness
that connects us all.

> When going looks like coming back,
> The clearest road is mighty dark.[13]
>
> —Lao-tzu

The oneness is the individual qualities that make us who we are. Why we are different from the next person. Person—how our particular cells are organized for
thought, and action. When a human being is born he is not fully developed. The

Illus. 43

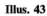
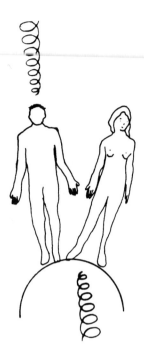

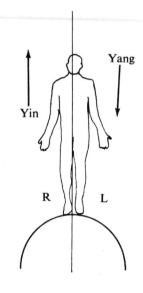

Yin

Yang

R   L

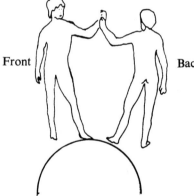

Front   Back

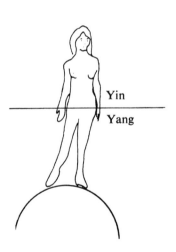

Yin

Yang

Illus. 44

A   B

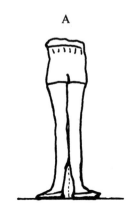

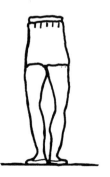

brain-nerve channels develop different patterns for speech, behavior, and thought. This depends upon our genes, cultural environment, and food.

But our oneness is also the sameness that connects us all. We have the same amount of body parts as a child or as a Nobel prize winner. We all need to take in food, drink, and air; we take what we need and get rid of the waste.

Jesus said, "If those who lead you say to you: 'See the kingdom is in heaven,' then the birds of the heaven will precede you. If they say to you: 'It is in the sea,' then the fish will precede you. But the kingdom is within you and it is without you. If you will know yourselves, then you will be known and you will know that you are the sons of the living Father. But if you do not know yourselves, then you are in poverty and you are poverty.[14]

—The Gospel According to Thomas

Classification II

All things bear the shade on their backs
And the sun in their arms;
By the blending of breath
From the sun and the shade,
Equilibrium comes to the world.[15]

—Lao-tzu

In the body it is easy to see the two divisions: front body–back body, flexor–extensor, upper and lower (Illus. 43).

In Oriental diagnosis there are two major divisions for body types.

Yin structure: long and narrow bone structure and features, large eyes, tall, thin build, rounded shoulders, long limbs, more mental abilities, soft muscles. A yin person may need to do more yang, active sequences to experience wholeness, and eat food with more yang components.

Yang structure: short and wide bone structure and features, small deep-set eyes, solid or stocky build, square shoulders, shorter limbs, physical abilities, tighter muscles. A yang person may need to do more yin relaxing sequences to experience wholeness, and eat food with more yin components.

The first comprehensive book on dance technique to appear in printed form was written by Carlo Blasis (1803–1878), a well known and highly respected Italian dancer. In the first chapter he puts dancers into two categories. The first is knock-kneed, forming a triangle between feet and knees. The form is more contracted (yang) and the mobility is less active (yin) (Illus. 44A).

The second he calls "bandy-legged," the lower limbs forming a bow shape. The form is more expanded (yin) and mobility is more active (yang) (Illus. 44B).

He explains in great detail the difference in training needed for these two types. The first must try to separate the parts that are too close together while the second must concentrate on bringing the parts that are separated closer together. The knock-kneed dancer has greater delicacy of movement (yin), but the bandy-legged dancer has more strength and elevation (yang).

All traditional cultures, recognizing that physical phenomena has two directions, created symbols to express them (Illus. 45, 46, and 47).

Illus. 45

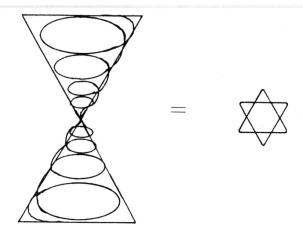

Illus. 46

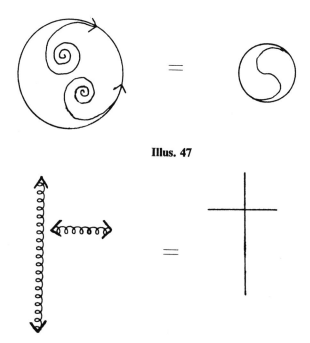

Illus. 47

Classification III

The way begot one,
And the one, two:
Then the two begot three
And three, all else.[16]

—Lao-tzu

In *Ayurveda,* the medicine of India, the human constitution is divided into three types based on the five basic elements of water, earth, fire, air, and ether. These three *tridosha* are responsible for individual preferences, temperaments, emotions, and body functions.

1.   *Vata is the combination of air and ether.*   It is the subtle energy that governs biological movement. People of this constitution are often physically underdeveloped, either too tall or too short, have dry and kinky hair and have prominent joints. They are creative, alert and restless and often sleep less than other types. They have quick mental understanding, but may also tend toward being nervous and anxious. The diagonal series in Chapter 5 is recommended for this type, to free the head and arms.

2.   *Pitta is the combination of fire and water.*   This governs metabolism, digestion, and body temperature. These people are medium height with a yellowish complexion and have thin hair. They usually have good digestion, strong appetites and warm body temperature. They are sharp and intelligent but may tend toward anger and jealousy. They are ambitious and often financially well-off. Sequences in Chapter 5 that free the torso are recommended.

3.   *Kapha is the combination of water and earth* (Illus. 48).   This lubricates joints, heals wounds and gives vigor and stability. These people often have dark hair, well-developed bodies, bright complexion, thick skin and often excess weight. They have good stamina and are generally happy, calm, and loving but they may tend toward greed or possessiveness. Sequences in Chapter 5 that free the hip sockets are recommended.

Illus. 48

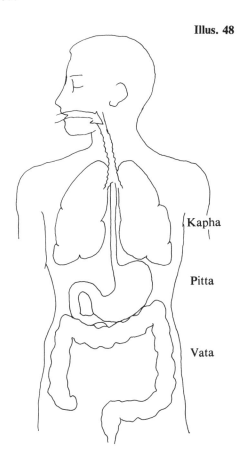

Kapha

Pitta

Vata

Kapha—water and earth
Pitta—fire and water
Vata—air and ether

Classification IV

Rudolph Steiner saw four types of individuals. He called these types "the four temperaments" and based them on the laws of the four elements of earth, water, air and fire.

In the *melancholic* he drew characteristics from the earthly element. Like a rock, the weight of the earth is felt. The face is pale and the eyes are dreamy, the shoulders sloping, the bones prominent and the skin is thin. The melancholic enjoys quiet activities, painting, drawing or poetry and usually does not like to become involved in sports or does not enjoy energetic games. There is often much clarity, precision and structure in this temperament. He may be likened to a geode which, when broken open, reveals a crystal inside. Propulsion or partner sequences are recommended. Excess refined sugar and dairy foods are to be avoided.

The *phlegmatic* temperament is based on the element of water: the fluid with the many changing states, from the raging sea to the dew on the morning grass. The body is often a little bit chubby while the eyes are peaceful and happy. The personality is adaptable and often refreshing to others. Because there is so much fluid movement in the body affecting digestion, the phlegmatic is often deeply involved with food. This temperament is inclined to stick to the familiar and does not venture too far into the unknown. Spatial tension sequences are recommended. Overeating should be avoided.

The *sanguine* temperament is the manifestation of air. It is shaped by everything and is constantly moving and adjusting and causing movement of others. Held in one place too long it becomes stale, or bottled up. The sanguine is optimistic, humorous, and light, with senses that are strong and a creative spirit that is alive. He is interested in communication and may be likened to a little bird twittering from branch to branch. Awareness of the body in Chapter 5 is recommended. Spices and stimulants are to be avoided.

The *choleric* temperament displays the element of fire, capturing everyone's attention. The body often has compact muscles and a firmness in the face. The choleric may flare up like the "bossy one" or sit like burning coals, watching those around him. He is able to inspire, heal, and cleanse others through his guiding light. Breathing sequences are recommended. Excess fat or oil is to be avoided.

Classification V

In Oriental medicine the theory of the five phases was used for classifying people, colors, sounds, sensations, animals, emotions, and everything else. It is based on the five basic transformations or processes and is represented by the symbols: tree, fire, soil, metal, and water. It is important to remember that these are processes that are moving tendencies and not to be seen as static elements (Illus. 49).

The *tree* phase is associated with upward expanding motion, a growing phase, and a gaseous state. It corresponds to spring, green, anger, wind, and the sour taste. Pelvis and leg sequences are recommended.

The *fire* phase is maximum activity upward, very expanded, a plasmic state. It corresponds to summer, red, excessive joy, heat, and the bitter taste. Relaxation and breathing sequences are recommended.

Illus 49

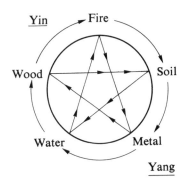

The outer arrows show the supporting cycle and the inner arrows show the controlling cycle.

The *soil* phase is coming back down to a balanced, neutral, or semi-condensed state. It corresponds to Indian summer, yellow, worry, damp, and the sweet taste. Awareness of total body is recommended.

Metal represents functions in declining and gathering to a solidified state. It corresponds to autumn, white, sadness, dry, and the pungent taste. Partner sequences are recommended.

Water is the floating or melting state after resting and before activity begins. It corresponds to winter, black, fear, cold, and the salty taste. Spatial tension and propulsion sequences are recommended.

Classification VI
Six Senses

Most people have a sense dominance—some are stimulated to move or learn by seeing, others by hearing and others by feeling. Yin is a wider scope or dimension, less stimulus, and shorter waves of vibration. Yang is a narrower scope or dimension, stronger stimulus, and longer waves of vibration.

1. *Touch is the most yang sense*—most direct (Illus. 50).
2. *Taste is less yang*—one can taste by many liquid experiences (Illus. 51).
3. *Smell—least yang.* We can smell many aromas in the air (Illus. 52).

Illus. 50

Illus. 52

Illus. 51

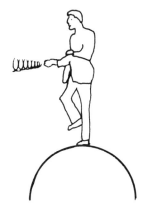

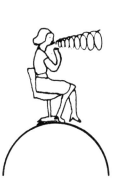

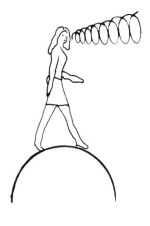

Illus. 53

Illus. 54

Illus. 55

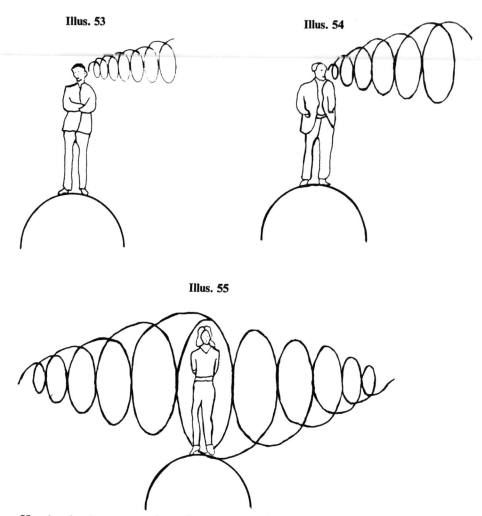

4. *Hearing is yin*—we can hear from a great distance by spiral vibration waves (Illus. 53).

5. *Seeing—more yin.* We can see so much. Even when we close our eyes we still see visions, lights, and more (Illus. 54).

6. *Kinesthetic—most yin.* We can sense many things. We have a feeling about this or that based on no special reason (Illus. 55).

Classification VII
Seven Levels of Movement

The stimulus for movement may come from many places.

1. *Mechanical.* During the nine months in the womb, we never made any conscious decisions to form organs, etc. After birth, we breathe, our organs work, and blood flows. Any activity we do every day, we don't have to think about. It becomes automatic. This makes our lives easier. We could not function if we had to control every move. The Dervish dances are an example.

2. *Sensory.* We begin to taste, touch, smell, hear and see, and this stimulates our movement. We are hungry so we move to get something to eat. Those senses

personally interpreted as feelings move us to many dances. Fertility rites are an example.

3. *Sentimental.* The emotions rule. We are sad so we stand or move a certain way. Or so happy we walk briskly or "jump for joy." Much modern dance expresses movement stimulated by emotions. Using this principle we can often change our moods by changing the way we move.

4. *Intellectual.* We begin to learn that certain muscles should be stretched or our cardio-vascular system "needs" toning up to function well. Our intellect dictates, not our feelings. "I think I should jog today"—the media tells us, "no pain, no gain." Many dances tell stories, teach, or pass down traditions.

5. *Social.* Society moves in this direction, and I want to be part of society so I move this way. Everybody is going to the prom, so I will go too. The popular social dances reflect the thinking, ideas, social taboos, and customs of the times. Folk and popular dances reflect this.

6. *Ideological.* We begin to think from a larger perspective, including universal movement. We observe the process of change (movement) from a perspective that never changes (stillness). This view with a broader scope affects our movement. This movement alters our perceptions and self expression. I share this change through daily life or performing. The Alexander Technique reflects this by learning to stop the habitual ego response and using the governing reflex to stimulate movement. Spiritual exercises in meditation, breathing, body control, and yoga, when done with awareness, were intended to remain in this class.

7. *Supreme.* Total conscious awareness allowing heaven and earth and the spiral to move you. Any and all movement totally present in the moment. No technique or style can train or teach this. It just is.

Each of us moves in all these ways and jump from one mode to another without thinking.

Classification VIII

The Chinese have developed a study of the art of face reading called *Siang Mien*. Through this one can understand a person's given natal character tendencies. Face shapes are divided into eight categories based on the eight trigrams of the I Ching:

1. *yin—moon shape:* round with curves and lacking prominent bone structure. Drink less and eat foods with minerals. Spatial tension series recommended.

2. *yin—jade face:* prominent cheek bones while narrow at the top and bottom. Eat more leafy greens. Arms series recommended.

3. *yin—tree face:* has more length than width throughout the forehead, cheekbones, and jaw. Eat more whole grains and beans. Pelvis and leg series recommended.

4. *yin and yang—earth face:* a wide, square jaw and narrower forehead. Eat more sea vegetables. Propulsion series recommended.

5. *yin and yang—fire face:* wide forehead, high cheekbones and a narrow, long chin. Eat more root vegetables. Spiral in legs series recommended.

6. *yang—wall or iron face:* square shape and strong bone structure. Eat softer foods (noodles). Relaxing series recommended.

7. *yang—bucket face:* a wide forehead with a slight taper. Eat more vegetables. Partner series recommended.

8. *yang—king face:* bony and prominent forehead, cheekbones and jaw. Chew your food more. Breathing series recommended.

There are irregular faces where one side is very different from the other in one or more features. For this the diagonal series is recommended.

Classification IX

One ancient type of astrological classification is called the nine star ki cycle. It is based on the nine planets or the nine constellations over the north pole, where vibrational influence on the earth is strong. To calculate your natal year number, add the last two digits until you reduce to one digit and then subtract from ten for the 1900s, from eleven for the 1800s, and so on. Note that the new year begins February 5, not January 1. A person born in 1978 is a four, born in 1945, a one.

Number nine is the most expanded, like fire. People born in this year are active, outgoing, sociable and happy. Manifest in the head.

The number eight is soil. These people are serious, orderly, deep thinkers with intelligent character. Manifest in the left leg.

Number seven is metal. They have strength and logic and are the most practical. They tend to be strong in common sense and everyday matters but also enjoy socializing. Manifest on right side of torso.

Number six is also metal. These people have an inwardly directed character and are concerned with ethical and orderly behavior, with a strong will and faith. Manifest in right leg.

Number five is balanced earth in the center. They have a clear, well-defined character and often become the center of any relationship. Manifest in the center of the torso.

Illus. 56

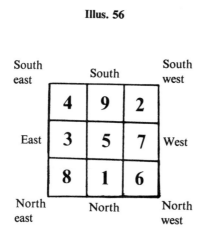

Illus. 57

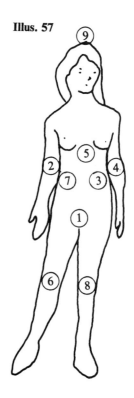

Numbers four and three are both wood. Threes are more aesthetic, brilliant, outgoing and active. Manifest on left side of the torso. Fours are more mature, thoughtful, dependable and ambitious. Manifest in left arm. Both are emotional and poetic.

Number two is soil. These people are outgoing and social with a lot of nurturing and teaching energy. Manifest in right hand.

Number one is water. These people are easy-going, agreeable, adaptable, and creative. Manifest in lower torso. Sequences are recommended under the five transformations (see Classification V).

Classification X

Kabbalah is the tradition of Jewish mysticism. The *En-sof* (E=without, sof=end) is the name for God, which symbolizes total unity beyond comprehension. From this, ten lights or *sefiroth* spring forth. They are abstract entities through which all change takes places. A person may perceive one of the manifestations or several as being dominant in himself. The aim is to become capable of seeing all the parts and their functions in unison in the world, as well as in one's self.

1. *Kether:* crown, unit—head
2. *Hokhmah:* wisdom—brain

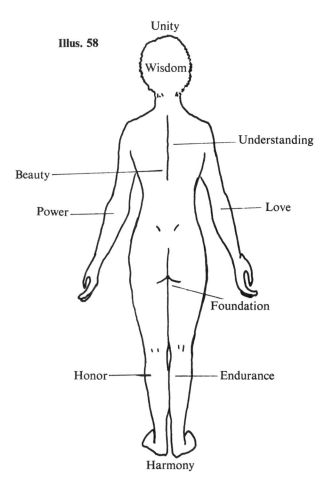

Illus. 58

3. *Binah:* intelligence and understanding—heart
4. *Hesed:* mercy and love—right arm
5. *Gevurah:* judgment or power—left arm
6. *Tifereth:* beauty—chest
7. *Netsah:* victory and endurance—right leg
8. *Hod:* glory and majesty (honor)—left leg
9. *Yesod:* foundation—genital organs
10. *Malkuth:* harmony and completeness—feet

These attributes can be contacted by attention to the corresponding body part (Illus. 58).

This is similar to Indian *mudras* (postures) used to convey an idea.

Classification XI

Listed are eleven planetary currents of energy patterns that influence all phenomenon. Movement can be initiated or supported by these flow patterns (Illus. 59).

Illus. 59

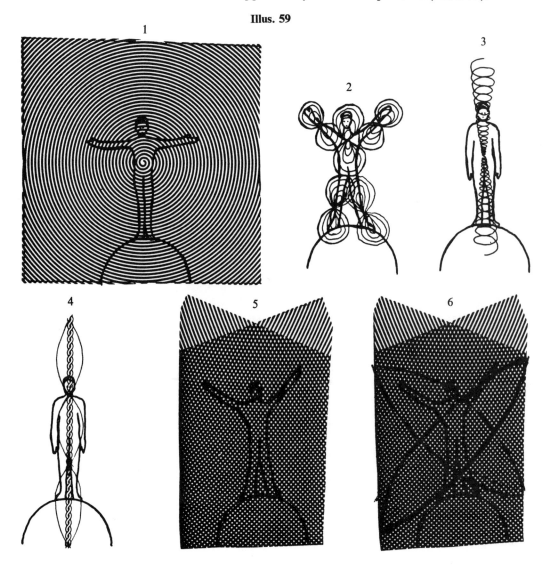

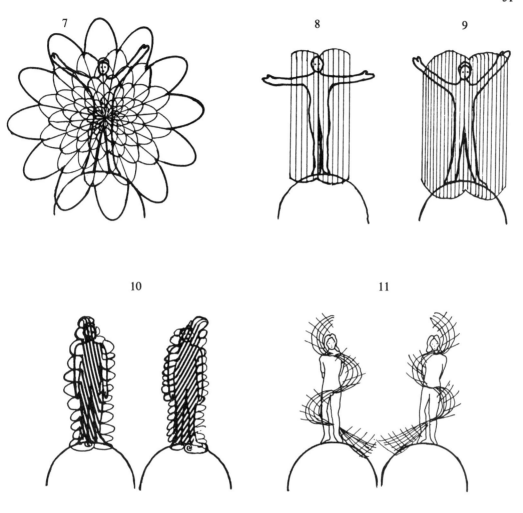

51

1. infinite to infinitesimal spiral (and back)
2. figure eight or pattern of infinity
3. spiral from above and below
4. double helix
5. simple "x" or diagonal
6. double "x" or diagonal
7. chrysanthemum or comet path (expand-return center)
8. twelve meridians
9. twenty-four meridians
10. meridians twisted right and left
11. crossed serpentine right and left

Classification XII

The twelve astrological classifications are:
January 21–February 19: Aquarius—tiger—1986—legs, ankles, blood system.
February 19–March 20: Pisces—rabbit—1987—feet, lymphatic system.

March 20–April 20:   Aries—dragon—1988—head, cerebrospinal system.

April 20–May 20:   Taurus—snake—1989—neck, throat, cerebellum and ears.

May 20–June 21:   Gemini—horse—1990—nerves, lungs, hands, arms and shoulders, tubes.

June 21–July 22:   Cancer—sheep—1991—chest cavity, breasts, stomach and mucous membranes.

July 22–August 22:   Leo—monkey—1992—heart and spine.

August 22–September 23:   Virgo—rooster—1993—solar plexus, spleen, food metabolism.

September 23–October 23:   Libra—dog—1994—kidneys, belt at navel level.

October 23–November 22:   Scorpio—boar—1995—sex organs, excretory functions.

November 22–December 21:   Sagittarius—rat—1996—pelvic region, sciatic nerve, hips, the muscular system, locomotion.

December 21–January 21:   Capricorn—ox—1997—skeleton, skin, knees and joints.

Note that the years for the animals begin February 4, not January 1. The tiger year is February 4, 1986 to February 4, 1987. To determine your animal year of birth count back from the dates given.

This chart may be used in many ways. If you are a Leo you may have a lot of activity centered around the heart so that you may want to choose a process that would disperse it or spread it out. Or you may find that you do not have enough energy around the heart and you may want to choose a process to develop that part of yourself.

Illus. 60

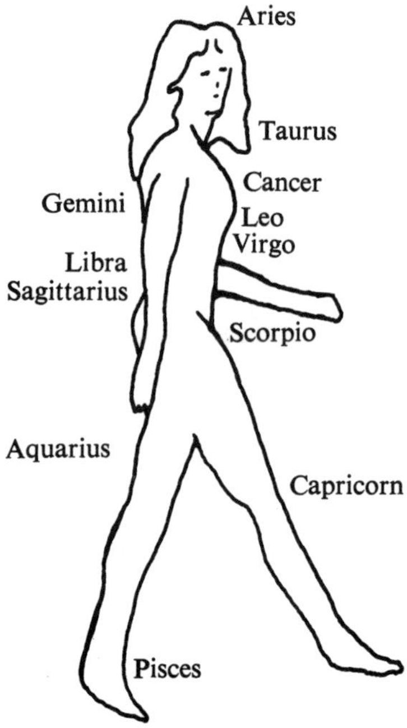

We see that most cultures categorize the many billions of people in these two to twelve classifications or types. Notice your tendency or type and choose the appropriate sequences. Different types of people will need different types of activity to center themselves. A water person will often need a more grounding type of process to balance that floating quality. A floating quality is not necessarily "bad," but we should not be stuck in any one movement style. A metal or heavier person would need to practice light and airy movements to offset the tendency to sink down and gather in. More food and thought recommendations will be given later as a vehicle for change.

2. History of Dance and Man's Relationship to Motion in the Body

"Anyone can do what I do if he does what I did."
—F. M. Alexander[1]

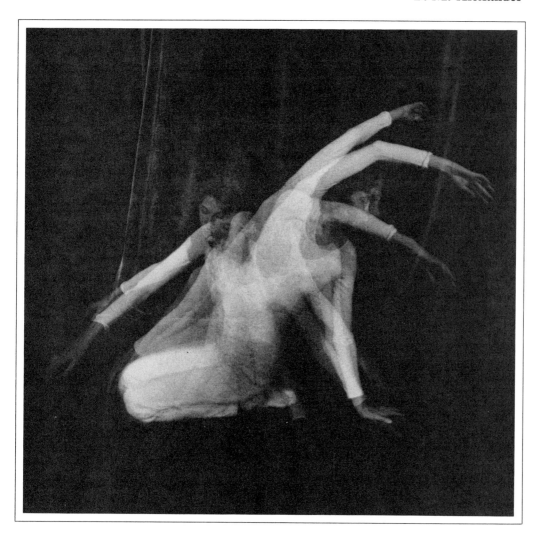

1. History

Every epoch in history on every part of this globe developed its own dance images and idioms through which people expressed themselves. Dance changes according to climate, religious beliefs, diet, codes of morality, and even clothing. From earliest times primitive man danced around in a circle (or spiral) trying to become one with the universal energy. To appease the gods, to give thanks, to ask for rain, to communicate with the divine or tell stories, dance or movement was used.

Dancing—what is it? An arrangement of patterns in space, an arrangement in time, or rhythm in the audible and visible sphere. It moves, excites, compels, or persuades us. With close physical sympathy, danger contracts us while a free floating leap expands us. Pattern, form, symmetry, asymmetry, distortion, stylization, gesture, and expression of human feeling are all included. Gestures are the same in many parts of the world. Many of the East Indian and Japanese dance gestures correspond to American Indian sign language.

Why dance—what was it for?

Either religion, or magic, or teaching, or entertainment. Early man worshipped natural forces, thunder, moon, sun, rain and animals. Primitives believed that if they acted out something and said proper magical words they could make it happen. Dancer priests passed down all information, moral training and ethics, history, wisdom and the rules for health, conduct and behavior through dance and song. On the island of Gaua, in New Hebrides, old men stood with bows and arrows and shot dancers who made mistakes.

Dance was used to heal through medicine men and to destroy through voodoo or black magic. It was used as a fertility ritual for agriculture as well as humans. After great disasters such as the Black Death and the French Revolution, widespread dance crazes followed. The whole population gave itself unconsciously and quite spontaneously to a kind of fertility ritual to rebuild.

Almost all primitive people have war dances to work up fighting spirit, excitement, and courage. Socrates said, "The best dancer is also the best warrior."[2]

There are dances of skill. In Sumatra a maiden dances balancing three trays with lighted candles. In Tibet a spirit dancer works with ropes. In Mexico while dancing the *rebozo*, the dancer unties a knot in a sash with her feet on the ground. And in many parts of the East there are sword dances.

There were dances for birth and death. The Ju Ju of West Africa have a solemn ceremony to help the ghost of the dead. When one is killed in battle, the Fox Indians dance for an hour a day for 15 days and praise his heroic deeds to release his spirit. Dances of birth were usually joyful and thankful.

For children there are play dances and old rituals adapted and simplified, from the maypole dance to ring-around-a-rosy.

Later courtship dances were used to introduce boys and girls who were old enough to marry. In some primitive people, the gestures were restrained. In Samoa, the responses are made only with the eyes. Amongst other primitives the gestures were frenzied, verging on orgiastic. When dances become untraditional, they reflect a change in community life. "The Rumba, which when not dull was often vulgar, became a dance of allurement with subtly changing moods ranging from flirtation to passion but without a single suggestive movement."[3] The American social dance, ballroom and square dancing, are courtship dances.

Dance has been used to express aggression, competition and repression. Actions and feelings that were not allowed to be expressed openly were expressed through dance. Society and the underworld meet. In some cultures males and females were not allowed to touch, but the gap has closed in dance. Dance also emerges as a rebellion to present conditions.

Dance became theater and entertainment when the dancer performed not for his own benefit, but for the audience.

So we can see there are many reasons for dance in recorded history. In my opinion dance movement started with humans first trying to recreate the physical, psychological and spiritual energies which are connected with the force of the infinite universe. Then they tried to recreate the energy of the environmental elements. If water was needed, humans would make their body vibrate like water energy, floating, lateral, side to side. If heat or fire was needed they would vibrate their bodies like fire, darting in a vertical direction. All movement is a reflection of infinity and any "art" tries to contain the feeling of infinity and interpret it. This was later translated as paying homage to the gods.

One carry-over in dance worth nothing has been the custom of giving thanks—from the early days of ritual, where the whole dance was to give thanks, to now, a simple gesture. In Indian dance you thank the floor by stamping your foot on it before you dance. In ballet you always curtesy in thanks at the end of a lesson. Japanese *Noh Dance* is preceded with a bow of thanks. And even in ballroom dancing when the song finishes it is customary to clap in thanks.

Once we leave primitive dances which are similar throughout the world we can see dances growing out of area and location.

Western civilization idealized man and made the human body a crucible of energy. So dance became an expression of action, designed to show the causes of man's inner conflicts as they reflect his being. Eastern dances are enacted as a totality within a stable world which accepts conflict as basic to all human existence.

In the West in the Middle Ages, dance and drama were split from religion when the church split body and soul. In the East, dance never severed ties with religion. Oriental religious dance became gestural dance. By idolizing gods the Asiatics turned the human body into an instrument of gesture and symbol focusing on contemplation. When Eastern Dervishes turn, they close their eyes and find the point of stillness inside. When Western ballet dancers turn, they spot (find a point of stillness) outside of themselves.

In the West the individual put his personality into his dance. In the East the dances were shaped collectively, not showing the individual personality. In the West, love is shown for human male and female. In the East, the love is divine for God. In the West we conquer space and leap around a stage. In contrast to our aggressive approach, the Easterner is not space conscious but puts great emphasis on slight changes in expression.

2. East

Once the painter paints his picture on canvas, duality has arisen. We have the painter and the picture. The dancer has something unique. The unity is not broken: the dancer is the dance. God is not a painter who has painted the world. Otherwise he would be separate from it. God is a dancer. . . . He is it.[4]

"The whole body becomes so expressive that one might almost say the body is thought."[5] In India, according to Hindu legend all life began in heaven and the world was created by Lord Shiva "in a dancing mood." Ever since gods have danced and the dance was their great gift to man.

The hands have many gestures and there are set movements for all body parts, recorded in the *Natya Shastra*, the dancer's Bible. Throughout many invasions the dance has been preserved by temple dancers. *Kathakali* style told passion plays of Hindu legends. The Indian dancer did not put his own life in his body because it was thought that he would then miss the strength of the angels in posture and gesture. Over and over we see the idea of emptying oneself to receive the divine.

In Sri Lanka dances are rooted in ancient wisdom and traditional folk humor. The masked dancers have a gift for mimicry, combining realism and ritualism.

In Burma dance has always been the most popular art form. The technique is based on an early Burmese god-inspired mad woman who performed the stories. The body is characterized by a back that is curved, knees that are bent, and faces that are smiling.

The dances of Cambodia display extreme delicacy and dreamlike quality, while Siamese dances have more action.

In Java the audience is enlightened, not entertained. This dance form is famous for its slow movements and a swaying and spiraling rhythmic surge that creates a soothing quality.

In contrast, Balinese dance is impetuous and noisy, showing naiveté and innocent gaiety.

In the dances of the Philippines, the influence of foreign conquest is clearly seen, particularly Chinese, Indian, Arab, and Spanish. Because of the warm climate, the dances are characterized by an emphasis on the torso, vivid facial expression, inner intensity and mystic grace. With flowing movements of the arm, they generate a general playfulness.

In Hawaii the hula began as a dance of worship, man identifying with Nature. Breaking waves are shown in sensuous contractions of the body, the whole body playing and laughing.

Drama, dance and opera were one in China, with very stylized forms using props as symbols. Because the Chinese trained their bodies with such precision, they became the world's best acrobats and jugglers. They developed an eloquent gesture language to communicate, while keeping the spine straight, the steps small, and the head expressive but unobtrusive. In their dance the world of make-believe triumphs over the real. A dance of a girl stepping into a rocking boat, a ferry man rowing her across a lake, and helping her out, is performed without props.

The Koreans, as mountain people, hold their traditions through dances of fairies, demons and animal ghosts. Movements are elegant and costumes are colorful.

Until the end of World War II, Japanese court dancers were not seen outside the Imperial Palace. The *Bugaku*, which came from India, via Tibet and China to Japan, was the most popular form of entertainment at the royal court. A more acrobatic and comic form of the stately Bugaku appealing to the general public was called the *Sarugaku*, or monkey dance. Originating at ancient Shinto and Buddhist festivals, it was the first native dance of Japan.

The fifteenth century gave birth to the Japanese drama called No, or Noh. This highly symbolic and stylized theater precedes dancing with dialogue, music and singing. The style includes precise movements, exact expressiveness, erect stance, and sometimes masks.

Until the seventeenth century there was no popular theater for the unintellectual audience. *Kabuki* (*Ka*-song, *bu*-dance, *ki*-technique), an offshoot of *Noh*, was created in 1596 by O-kuni, a ritual dancer at the Shinto Shrine of Izumo. She danced to raise money for the shrine. Soon she added her own variations to Shinto-Buddhist dances. In time she was overtaken. Her desire to dance was stronger than her desire to serve the shrine, and kabuki was born.

A basic principle in Japanese dancing is a natural line of movement with no strain for form and a strong emphasis on stature. In 1912 a musical comedy department opened at the Imperial Theater in Tokyo, beginning the introduction of Western dance to Japan. Ballet and modern dances have since become quite popular.

3. Middle East

Three thousand years ago in the Middle East, a high culture developed in ancient Egypt, its dance comprising introvert (self-examining) and extrovert (performing) tendencies of movement. The Egyptians danced of nature, animals, dreams, tribes, and the death and resurrection of *Osiris*, their God. There were no social dances. The aristocrats whose lives are recorded in monuments did not participate in choral dance, nor couples, nor solo dance. The temple dancers are shown taking gentle steps with arms outstretched in rhomboid form, similar to a frozen motion picture, often called figure dances.

Many ceremonial temple dances or movements originated in ancient religions and continue today. Young girls were consecrated from an early age to the service of God. They lived in the temple from childhood and learned sacred dances. In the learning room there was a larger than life adjustable apparatus with inscriptions said to be 4,500 years old. As the figure was placed in different positions the young pupils stood before it to sense and remember the postures. Each posture had form and content.

The members of the sect knew the alphabet of these postures. When the elder priestesses performed the ritual of the day, the brethren read truths that were placed there thousands of years before.

With this their teachings were preserved and hidden from outside invasion. The dance movement concealed secrets of a particular sect.[6]

The Sufi sect is something like this today. You may work side by side with a member for five years and never know his beliefs. When and if he thinks you are ready he will tell you about the teachings and you may learn the language of their dance.

I think folk dances are a simplified version of these, expressing unity of a group of people. Folk dances were part of daily life and were often joyful, lively, and colorful, as in Israel.

In Spain the Eastern and Western cultures met and clashed. The dances were spread by gypsies. The word "gypsy" is a corruption of the word "Egyptian" but the gypsies were actually Indians, not Egyptians. The African Mohammedan, or Moors, settled by the thousands in Europe (612–1492). They inherited art and literature from the Persians. The Moorish dance had many characteristics of Oriental form to which they added African embellishments, including heavier shaking of the shoulders, rotation of the hips, snapping of the fingers and "muscle dancing."

A form of "muscle dancing" is practiced by all Mediterranean basin people, including Greeks, Armenians, Turks, Egyptians and Israelites. The dancers employ a lateral sliding of the neck back and forth on the shoulders. Later added to that the hips and shoulders remain quiet while the torso muscles jumped and rippled. What we call belly dancing is one example.

In 1492 the Moors were driven from Granada, their capital. Those who stayed behind combined Christian customs with their own, giving birth to classical Spanish dance, including the *fandango*, *bolero*, and *flamenco*. They all included complex rhythms, elaborate heel taps, and castanet patterns. Emotional relief was a driving force in Spanish dance. The gypsy men and women danced like tigers. Matched in strength and brilliance, they dance together but do not perform the same steps. These dance ideas were carried to South and Central America, Mexico, and to all Spanish colonies.

4. West

Primitive Greek Drama consisted of choruses and dances celebrating the death and rebirth of the god, *Dionysus*. The function was to warn, to teach morals, and to rouse and release the feelings. The gestures were stylized and dancers wore large masks so as to be seen at the back of the amphitheater. The dance was highly respectable with no violence or vulgarity. Harmony of line and dramatic power were accented.

The Romans, on the other hand, had a different opinion. Cicero said, "No sober person dances."[7] The average Roman had little inclination or aptitude for dancing. Because the dance was ecstatic, sober, realistically-minded Romans did not participate much. So they tended to imitate with pantomime and became extraordinary in this class. As the empire declined the Romans' respectability crumbled. Entertainment gave way to horror, brutality, dangerous acrobatics, and vile clowning. They often wore masks and became the forerunners of the *commedia dell'arte*.

In the East there is much variation from country to country. (Compare India and Japan, for example.) This is seen less in the West, but major changes can be seen over the years. (Compare traditional folk dances to break dancing.) In the East

(China) the traditional folk dances are still the dances of today. As countries become more "advanced," this changes.

The European and American continents' dancing seems to lead from folk dancing to ethnological and from social dancing onto the stage. Folk dancing grew out of the rituals of primitive man, encouraging the feeling of oneness or belonging to a certain group. Originally they were country or peasant dances that eventually spread to the cities because of their national and racial appeal. In folk dances geographical differences have caused some variations. Thus the dances of various mountain peoples are more closely related to one another than those of the people of the lowlands, although they may belong to the same country. Greeks, Italians, Russians, Poles, Americans, Frenchmen, Danes, etc., all have their own stylized folk dances.

Many ballets are based on folk dances; the English *Morris Dance* in Fokine's *Don Juan*; the Italian *Tarantella* in Bournonville's *Napoli*; gypsy dances in Massine's *Aleko*; and the list goes on, using the Polka, the Fandango, the Bolero, Minuet, or Jazz forms.

Through the centuries, dances undergo a similar process. An example would be the *Saraband* which originated in the Arabic Moorish or Persian tradition and came to the European courts through Spain. At an early period of its existence, it was considered wild and vile and even outlawed by the Spanish government. But as the dance spread, the European version was much calmer and polite. The minuet, the most popular social dance for 150 years, also began as a gay and lively dance. But in the Baroque and Rococo period in the French Court, the dance became static and unemotional to such a degree that Voltaire ridiculed it by saying, "They move without progressing a single step and end up on the very spot where they started."[8]

All dance steps emerge from the same physical mechanism using basic locomotor movements such as walking, running, hopping, skipping, sliding, galloping, or leaping. Most dances include some kind of turn, or whirl, or spin. Combined with certain characteristics of the environment (food, climate, terrain) and peculiarities of racial temperament (politics, customs, and the times) a particular dance is born.

Italy was the cradle of dance theater during the European Renaissance. Later the polished baroque beauty emerged from France. Music was important and the period was characterized by the madrigal (which stemmed from Gregorian chants), patterns of geometric design, color, and masks. The favorite dance of the fifteenth and sixteenth century was the *basse danse* which moved slowly and solemnly, feet never leaving the ground, in which dignity was always preserved. Again, as we have previously seen, a quiet dance is often followed in popularity by an active dance. In this case it was the *Saltarello* or tarantella, a gay dance with occasional leaps. Other dances of the eighteenth century were the minuet, gavotte, jig, and allemagne, which led to the waltz, polka and mazurka.

In the second half of the eighteenth century, bored with the minuet, people turned to the waltz, which seems to have originated in the mountain regions of Southern Germany and Austria. In the beginning it was considered vulgar and lewd because of its intoxicating rhythm, closeness of position, and joyful, almost ecstatic expression. The waltz was the most symbolic expression of the bourgeoisie, outliving the quadrille and the cancan.

These dances, along with many others laid the foundation for what is called "ballet" today. The word "ballet" derives from *balletti*, a diminutive for *balli*, a term for livelier dances. Although born in Northern Italy, theatrical ballet dancing came of age in France. In the next two hundred years as clothes became lighter, manners more refined, and dueling more expert, the ballet grew. All courtiers took dance lessons every day and took great pride in the coordination of arms and hands in counter rhythm to the feet. The postures and attitudes were noble and controlled, affected yet elegant, ornate, swift, and commanding. The ballet spread to many countries: Italy, France, England, Russia, America, and continents throughout the world. There were many great ballet dancers, teachers, and choreographers.

Vaslav Nijinsky was one of the greatest dancers of this age. He jumped high in the air and descended like a feather. It was like a miracle. Spectators and scientists were mystified. What he did is not supposed to be physically possible because of the gravitational force of the earth. When Nijinsky was asked, "How do you manage it?" he said, "That I cannot say because when it happens *I* am not there. I have tried to manage it and I have always failed. Whenever I try to manage it, it doesn't happen."[9]

In Cuba when Castro came to power he contacted Alicia and Fernando Alonso, two Latin dancers who had studied ballet thoroughly in America, and offered them carte blanche to establish a school and company in Cuba. With the blending of the two civilizations, the European and the Latin, African Cuban Folkloric subjects joined the characters in the classics. Ballet became so popular that Alicia Alonso became the First Lady of the country.

Music hall dancing was popular toward the end of the nineteenth century. One of the most famous was the French cancan. In the United States we had the Broadway theater, home of the later famous musicals. The forerunners were the Negro minstrel shows, which came straight off the plantations and into the dance halls. Participants did not think or theorize: they danced. Jazz and tap dancing followed, characterized by loose knees and ankles, snapping fingers, and a big smile. This was quite opposite to the ballet which had straight knees and highly controlled moves.

The turn of the century brought Isadora Duncan (1878–1927), an American dancer who threw off her corset and shoes and stripped dance of all needless ornamentation. She tried to clear away the accumulated debris of six hundred years of artificiality. She saw dance as a form of worshipping nature, reversing two thousand years of frivolity. She preached basics: dress sensibly, move freely, keep healthy, and consider yourself no one's slave. She excited the crowds in Europe and America. Her revolution was the basis for all modern dance today.

Modern dance styles in America today range from the crisp, linear, precise Merce Cunningham technique, to the spiral twists and deep emotional involvement of the Martha Graham technique, to the lighter, harmonious arcs of the Jose Limon or Eric Hawkins technique. Today the dances that are performed continue to be ballet, modern dance, and some outstanding folk groups (Russians or Israelites). The social dances are still whatever the food, environment, consciousness, and government dictate and permit.

Since the early 1900s ballet appears to be trying to get up from the earth and portray the image of weightlessness, while modern dance is closer to the floor, acknowledging the weight of the body. Much ballet has become a matter of technical brilliance (how many pirouette turns can a dancer do?), while modern dance often presents human predicaments and searches for solutions. But a renewal for spirit in dance seems to be lacking.

5. Eurythmy

Many believe this gap was filled by Rudolf Steiner in 1912 with the birth of eurythmy. He was not concerned with any kind of synthesis of contemporary trends but saw dance as having spiritual origin, drawing creative force and impulse from this. Steiner and Isadora Duncan were developing their art in the same place, Munich, Germany. But while Duncan strove to revive the classics, Steiner aimed to spiritualize the arts anew. With the coming of war many dance centers moved from Germany to Switzerland (Dalcroze, Laban, and Steiner).

In modern dance as taught by Rudolf Laban (the father of modern dance in Europe), the space that you dance in is limited to the reach of your kinesphere, bounded by the finger tips in every direction. But for the eurythmist there is no limit to space. There is the polarity of the centrifugal and the centripetal forces, creating endless space to be used. The movement in the soul is thinking, feeling, and willing. In the body, the movement is from: 1) the head and nervous system (the physical basis of thinking; 2) the rhythmic system of pulse and breath (the physical basis for feeling; and 3) the limb system (the physical basis of will).

In most types of dancing, movement is centered in the hips. In eurythmy it is the arms that give man the free experience of total space. From the horizontal they can reach upward or downward or balance in the middle.

Steiner believed that to acquire a pure conception of the quality of movement, one must study the sounds of speech, for every sound of speech is actually an invisible gesture in the *etheric* sphere (the sphere of the forces of life). He thought that most dance steps were already combinations of these sounds. It is like paraphrasing a piece of poetry into words and then the "poetry" is gone.

Vowels express inner feelings, while consonants express the outer world. Some sound gestures—L, M, and R—have no beginning and no end while explosive sounds such as B, D, P, G, and K have definite boundaries. The vowel sound "ah" produces a movement of the arms which opens them out to wide spaces. R is a continuous rolling gesture while T expresses a certain finality.

Everything is then carried into music, seeking to express the music itself and not just the subjective reaction to it. Sound in musical scales begins in the collar bone, extending to the upper arm, lower arm, wrist, and out through the hand. The form and flow of melody is brought to visible expression.

Steiner also used the experience of color as a means of conveying movement. The arms in the central position of the horizontal express green, the central color of the spectrum. When the arms bend in a downward or inward arc, they express more blue or purple. On the other hand, when the arms reach with palms up, an arc of levity, they express yellow to orange to red.

Eurythmy today is used to educate and to heal, drawing its inspiration and force from the spiritual world. In his quest for freedom, man has somehow lost his connection with the divine. "The art of eurythmy is one of the channels through which the spirit is again revealing itself to human consciousness. It is a path through which man may again find a way to that self-knowledge which is also a knowledge of the universe."[10]

This is part of a growing stream of teachings that are removing the power and control of the habitual ego personality and teaching one to exist within a larger framework. It is a logical progression from "I want to control" my body movements. Let us see this with "spiral thinking." We want to bypass the habitual ego from controlling movement, yet we can only use the self, which is partially that habitual ego, to do it. Tommy Thompson once gave a lecture on the "Fallacy of Self Improvement Techniques Using the Self You've Got."[11]

The technique, created by Frederick Matthias Alexander after many years of observing human movement, presents a landmark in the history of motion. Now movement is trained, not to be dictated by the individual or ego or body type, nor by emotions, senses, or habitual patterns, but by the reflexes. There is no set goal or position, yet ease in movement is achieved. It is not a learning, but an unlearning. A teaching not of something to do, but of something to allow.

6. Alexander's Discovery

Alexander's declared wish in writing the book *Man's Supreme Inheritance* (1910) was to show that "every man, woman and child holds the possibility of physical perfection; it rests with each of us to attain it by personal understanding and effort."[12] Conditions of misuse often precede and accompany defective functioning of the human mechanism. According to Alexander, human instinct has not developed at the same rate as man's inventive capacity. So we rely on instinctive guidance and control that is not geared to our rapidly changing environment. Man is unable to adapt himself quickly enough to the changes in civilization. Early man was forced day by day to make use of his mechanism by securing food and drink and by protecting himself from his adversary. With this came a correct use of his psycho-physical organism as a whole.

Today we leave out many steps in the life process. We call this advancement, or making life easier. But there seems to be a price to pay. Man's instinct has become an inadequate guide, especially in conditions of modern civilization. He depends on faulty or unreliable guidance for his psycho-physical mechanism to operate. This, of course, leads to further misuse, strain, and eventually to a state of involuntary tension and fatigue, where behavior is only a reaction and not a conscious response. Gradually what is wrong comes to feel right in the individual and the world.

After World War II Alexander hoped that the atomic bomb shocked the world enough to stop and realize that salvation lay in learning to "bridge the gulf between conscious and subconscious control of reaction." Knowing how to stop, refusing to give consent to habitual reaction, is the basic means for this change. He thought it was the only reliable means by which man could avoid "emotional gusts" which displayed prejudice, greed, jealousy, hatred, and the like, and destroyed the path for conditions of peace in the world.

The Alexander Technique does not set out to teach good posture, does not manipulate body parts, does not promise health and curing of aches and pains, and does not teach how to "hold" your self in a correct position. It is a process of reeducation by which you train yourself first to become aware of what you are doing. Then, in learning how not to reinforce reactive habitual behavior patterns, stereotyped responses are gradually eliminated. These habitual responses, a form of direct control, only serve to strengthen the ego, which prevents you from seeing yourself as part of a larger whole or environment. The technique utilizes indirect control with no direct interference with the workings of muscle groups.

Raymond Dart said, "We have the self and the 'not self' or environment that surrounds it, and that is the world or universe, of which each individual self forms such an utterly fragmentary part."[13]

Language creates barriers when trying to convey the Alexander Technique. Altering the dualistic thinking of body and mind was of concern to Alexander. He chose to call these two aspects of the single entity "the self." People of his time and even now regard their physical bodies as entities separate from their mental souls and their spirits. Our thinking process is constantly analyzing and then trying to reconstruct the whole. This is impossible.

F.M. Alexander was born in Tasmania, an island near Australia, on January 20, 1869. He grew up on a farm the eldest of eight children, and was involved in raising horses, an interest he never lost. As he grew older he chose acting and reciting Shakespeare as a career. As his career was developing he began to have trouble with his throat and he would lose his voice by the end of a recitation. The medications prescribed by the doctor did not help. The doctor told him not to use his voice and he would not lose it. This worked, of course, but did not solve his problem. He did notice that in daily conversation his voice was fine but when he recited he would lose it. This led him to a very important idea which he later phrased "use affects function"—how we use our bodies determines how they function.

So he spent the next ten years exploring the possibilities of his misuse and experimenting with ways to change. He discovered by his awareness that as he was reciting he pulled his head back and down, sucked in breath and depressed his larynx. With these interferences went a tendency to lift his chest and hollow his back, thus shortening his stature. It seems that the problem could be easily solved by just not doing these things and doing the right thing. But that is not as simple as it may seem. As F.M. Alexander was discovering, our senses are unreliable. What we think we are doing and what we are doing are often two different things.

For example, ask a friend to move his head without moving his shoulder. He thinks that he has succeeded. If you watch him, you will clearly see that his shoulders *have* moved. In that observation it is the kinesthetic sense that is unreliable. *Kinesthetic* perception deals with sensations of position and movement, heaviness and lightness, holding or freeing. For example, when you stand with arms by your side and look straight ahead and then move your hand, you know that your hand is moving even though you are not looking at it. That is your kinesthetic sense.

The reason that we have "faulty sensory appreciation" with the kinesthetic sense may be explained like this: the kinesthetic sense works partly through the muscle spindles in the muscles. These spindles are tiny mechanisms whose function is to convey information from muscles to higher centers in the brain about the state of muscles and then receive information back from the brain as to what to do about it. But if a muscle is in a prolonged contractive state the feedback system of the spindles does not work optimally. So we cannot feel what we are doing but, of course, we do not know it.

So F. M. Alexander experimented with mirrors to get visual information. He realized that his response to the thought of reciting was a total pattern of misuse beginning with the head. He had discovered what was causing his vocal trouble. Usually when something is wrong we think we must do something to change it. But he realized that *doing* more only tangled him more. The only solution that worked was to first stop doing what he was doing the way he was doing it. This was a revolutionary contribution to human behavior and reaction. This principle distinguishes the Alexander Technique from any other "body corrective teaching." There is no teaching a "right way," only how to unlearn a wrong doing through awareness, inhibition, conscious control, and direction.

He found that he was able to maintain good use until the last second before the movement. At that moment he went back to his familiar and comfortable use. This is the critical moment—the space between stimulus and response—the space within which the possibility of freedom from habit is most likely to occur. It is within this moment that Alexander's concept of inhibition comes into play. By this he meant delaying the instantaneous response to stimulus: withholding consent to automatic reaction until one could carry out a response that maintained the integrative action of the whole organism. He kept his awareness on not allowing the habitual contractive patterns of movement to take over. He took his awareness away from trying to do it right, and focused on the "means whereby." This includes watching the relationship between the head, neck, and spine, and not focusing on the end or what he was trying to do. Because as soon as he would focus on the end (end-gaining), he would lose his "means whereby" and pull his head back and down and lose the integrity of the organism.

To facilitate this means he developed a set of "directions" or "orders" establishing what he called the primary control: 1) "Allow the neck to be free" to free the muscles in his neck and not overtense them; 2) "allow the head to free forward and up" so as not to pull it back and down [*note:* the head is to be directed forward and up, not *put* there]; 3) "allow the back to lengthen and widen," lengthening his spine so as not to arch and shorten it, and widen his back instead of pulling it narrow; 4) "allow the knees to free forward and away." These directions were to be given sequentially and simultaneously, "one after the other and all at once."[14]

Anyone learning to use this work must go through these steps in some way. F. M. said, "Everyone must do the real work for themselves. The teacher can show the way but cannot get inside the pupil's brain and control his reaction for him."[15] We cannot control the behavior of others, but we can control our reaction to it. For this reason the work sessions are done with the eyes open in relationship to the environment, for we are never without an environment. Closing the eyes may take us into a wonderfully peaceful world but at some time we must open them and respond to outer influences.

In the course of motor learning, sets are developed which are not the best preparation for the movement. In fact they often hamper the movement. Because the organism adapts readily, they come to feel right. We don't even notice them because once the stimulus to move is received, the attention is focused on the goal. Through his teaching experience of forty years Alexander found this to be almost universally true.

As a simple example, if you ask a student to walk, he will walk as he habitually knows. If you ask him to keep in mind the directions and allow one knee to release forward, he will have a different experience of walking. Because even as he thinks of walking the muscles are set in his habitual pattern.

In 1965, an arresting neurological fact came to light. Changes in electric potential take place in the nerve cells in the frontal lobes of human brains *before*, as well as during and after voluntary muscular movements. Two German neurologists (Deecke and Kornhuber) found that while an individual is thinking about carrying out an action, the action is being preceded by a slow negative wave occurring in the front region of the brain. Drs. Falconer and Walter affirmed that negative waves of this sort "precede and accompany every conscious, spontaneous, voluntary decision and action from deciding to walk or talk to starting and stopping your car. They have termed it "the expectancy wave."[16]

By stopping and inhibiting and giving direction during the expectancy wave, the habitual reaction may be circumvented.

F. M. Alexander realized that "nature does not work in parts but treats everything as a whole." It is necessary to re-educate the whole person for change. If a student came with a backache to be fixed, Alexander would not say, 'I will fix your backache.' Rather, he might say, 'Your use of your total mechanism has gone wrong. I can teach you to improve efficiency of your total mechanism. Once you learn this, your overall condition will change, which will raise the general level of health and check the formation of harmful habits.'

This is also applicable in the field of emotional response. Emotional disturbances immediately affect our state of tonus. When one learns to allow the muscles to lengthen and not contract further, when the stimulus is given the emotional response may not build to explosion. The time gap allows for a more rational decision. This behavior is not suppressing and not exploding and provides a comfortable alternative.

He made no guarantees for cures. The technique is educational and preventive, not curative. Yet cases of paralysis, asthma, colitis and more have disappeared after lessons. "Amongst them too emerged those who improved in elocution and carriage and also became better in health and relieved from habitual aches and pains."[17]

The technique provides the knowledge and freedom to change but there is no must or obligation. The training replaces rigid habits with flexible, constant choices of behavior and movement. Any technique that offers change must also offer self reflection and a means.

To offer just words or ideas for a better life is often not enough to budge us from our deep-set channels of habit.

Simply put, Alexander's technique brings about psychophysical change by teaching the individual to recognize and prevent habitual reactions which interfere with fundamental reflex patterns, that maintain the integrity of the whole organism. One learns to maintain "thinking in activity," as John Dewey called it. "The Alexander Technique is a method for improving motor performance by integrating the voluntary and reflex components of a movement in such a way that the voluntary does not interfere with the reflex and the reflex facilitates the voluntary."[18]

F. M. Alexander taught his brother, A. R. Alexander, to teach the technique. The two taught in England, America, and Australia. They taught such noted figures of the day as John Dewey, Aldous Huxley, George Bernard Shaw, and George E. Coghill.

George Coghill (1872–1941) was a noted biological scientist who did work on animal locomotion, correlating the development of behavior with the development of anatomical structure. After thirty years of study he said, "movement was integrated from the start, with the 'total pattern' of the head and trunk, dominating the 'partial patterns' of the limbs. In the total pattern of behavior there were two parts, 'one overt or excitatory and the other covert or inhibitory.' The inhibitory factor was essential for the successful execution of specific reflexes."[19]

Coghill's ideas supported Alexander's discoveries and gave them scientific basis. (Again, science and the practical agree.) The work of Rudolph Magnus and Sir Charles Sherrington also supported Alexander's work. Magnus said after years of animal research, "the whole mechanism of the body acts in such a way that the head leads and body follows."[20]

In my opinion, because F. M. Alexander is dead there is no "one style only" to teach his work. We are grateful to Marjory Barlow, Patrick MacDonald, Walter Carrington, Dr. Wilfred Barlow, and Marjory Barstow, who were trained by F. M. Alexander and have continued to teach the work for more than fifty years. What is called the "Alexander Technique" is a way of conveying through the hands the principles that F. M. Alexander discovered. These principles of the universe existed (as he knew) long before he did, and exist now after his death. They are uncovered and taught periodically by selected humans.

Summaries of F. M. Alexander's Discoveries:
1.   The dynamic relationship of the head to the neck to the torso is "the primary control" governing our physical body. This also applies to the animal kingdom. Watch a snake move. If the head is pulling down, the whole body has some manifestation of excess downward energy or contraction, and lacks spiralic supporting tensional balance throughout.

2.   "Means whereby." Our awareness stays with the process, the steps in between. In this case, the process is keeping the neck free instead of focusing entirely on our objective. Sole focus on our objective invariably makes us forget how we use ourselves to accomplish this.

For example, I want to reach over and pick up a book. If I think about the book I will most likely not be thinking about my neck being free, which would facilitate the head's tendency to maintain dynamic balance throughout. I have abandoned the awareness of myself for the desire to have the book, and have not yet reached the book. I find myself somewhere in between. Without the means whereby, I am not with myself, and not with the book, and because of this I am not totally present in the moment.

3.   Inhibition. There is no way to pull our heads up from above. It is also not

possible to push it up from below. If you contract any of the neck muscles to pull the head up, you are simultaneously pulling it down. We must *stop* contracting the neck muscles to *allow* the head to free forward and up. It is interesting to note that since we are made of electromagnetic energy in a vibratory field of waves, we are subject to much constant movement. The nervous system functions to stop, control, and direct this energy either voluntarily or involuntarily.

The general effect of the supra segmental structures in our central nervous systems, whether in fore-, mid-, or hind-brains, is to produce coordination and control of segmental reflexes by inhibiting useless muscular activities and substituting them with purposive movements. "It is likely that many of the functional interactions between cortex, basal ganglia, and thalmus are directed toward securing a greater inhibitory control of sensorimotor activities—the more synapses the greater the possibility for interaction and integration."[21]

4. What is use? Judith Kestenberg speaks of body attitude as "the somatic core of the body image which changes with each new developmental phase . . . the way the body is shaped, how it is aligned in space, how body parts are positioned in relation to one another and to the favored position of the whole body. Body attitude also denotes all the patterns and phrases of movement for which there is readiness at rest. In addition, it indicates the qualities of movement which, through frequent use, have left their imprint upon the body."[22] In the technique we speak a lot about use. What does that mean? How we are, think, feel, speak, and do everything. We use the self that we have to do it. When we are just standing we are usually pulling or holding muscles in a certain way that is familiar. Even though we *think* we are just standing still, on many levels we are doing this and that. We may call this use. Figure 1, Kuan Yin in a pose of royal ease, is an example of good use.

Fig. 1

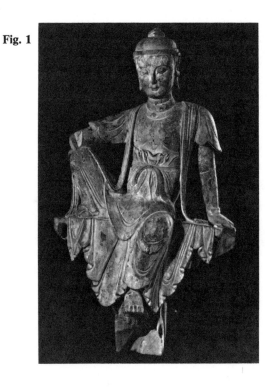

David Gorman presents these examples:

A.   Observe yourself holding a pen. It may actually weigh one ounce but we grasp on to it as if it weighed five pounds. We continue the misperception and tighten all the muscles in the arm and shoulder in order to write with five pounds, when the muscular activity sufficient to move the pen exists merely in our fingers. Where is the common sense? We are using ourselves not in accord with our design.

B.   We are at work and we get tired. Our choices would be: 1) to follow the instinct to lie down for a few minutes; or 2) to continue working and try to adjust our bodiesto it. Since we are at work we cannot lie down, so we adapt a sort of slouched down position (relaxed) and this becomes our tired response. Since this continues, the slouch becomes the way we use ourselves all the time. Then we go to bed and even when we wake up we are in tired response and so we are tired. The circle is endless but can be changed anywhere along the way.

*   *   *

Other ideas based on the principles of F. M. Alexander:

Frank Pierce Jones, a Professor of Classics at Brown University, was trained to teach the Alexander Technique by F. M. and A. R. Alexander. Once introduced to the technique for health reasons, Frank Jones decided to pursue Alexander's ideas, and was encouraged to do so by his wife, Helen. This meant uprooting his family (wife and three children) and his career for this unusual and revolutionary work. Lessons were expensive and they had to travel to get them. Yet through the combined efforts of this family, the work of Frank Jones has been a major contribution to the Alexander Technique. He taught and did research in the Greater Boston area for many years. His research and clarity on reflex responses demonstrated the technique scientifically and gave practical and sound reasons as to how and why the technique works.

There are two major reflex responses that take place in the body—attitudinal and righting. An example of the first is the startle reflex which occurs when the body must orient itself to some intrusion to its equilibrium. For example, a person encounters a loud sound. The body's response reacting to startle reflex is to pull the head back and down, pull the shoulders up, hollow the chest, and proceed to contract throughout the body. At this time, adrenalin is secreted. It is commonly known as the fight or flight reflex.

The other reflex response is called the righting reflex, which brings us back to our balanced relationship to gravity, a state of equilibrium or tensional balance, in which the head-righting plays the major role. If a horse falls and you hold his head down he will not be able to get up. If you allow the head to right itself, the body will follow by the anti-gravity muscles being activated.[23] The anti-gravity muscles, or the extensors, are a complete set of muscles that are designed to take us away from gravity.

As can be seen, the head-neck-body reflexes control deviation from normal upright stance as well as the return to it. The problem is that modern life often throws us into a startle or attitudinal (an attitude appropriate for the moment) pattern, but we never fully return from it, back to a freer state of existence. These held physical attitudes develop slowly and build on each other. It gets harder and harder to return

Fig. 2A

Fig. 2B

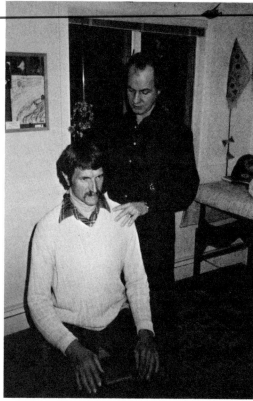

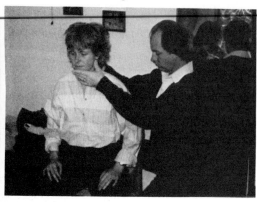

Fig. 3

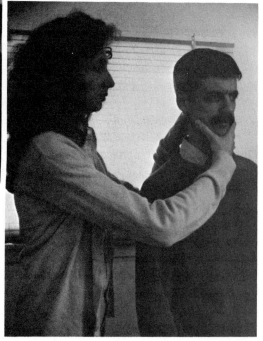

to a freer state of existence. When a pattern develops slowly, we do not notice it. So it feels right. In any kind of movement this greatly restricts our field of motion and often produces injury. Your conceptual brain has decided that your body will make a certain movement, but because of the build-up of tension creating unfree relationships between the parts, the movement is not possible. So frustration, injury, and sickness follow. The technique gives the individual the freedom to choose a response. Figures 2A and B show Tommy Thompson teaching. Figure 3 is the author.

Posture

Those who are bound by desire see only the outward container.[24]

—Lao-tzu

Is my posture correct? Am I standing straight?

These questions are pondered by many people. What is posture? Can there be a static position that is correct this moment and still be correct for tomorrow? Of course not. The earth has rotated two million times, the stars have moved, the planets have whirled by. How can we expect ourselves to have not moved in relationship to these? And what is supposed to be straight? The spine? It is curved already. Our heads should be straight? What does that mean?

Our bodies do not have a monitoring system that tells us when our posture is good and straight or not. Many people are hunched over or twisted in one way or another but they feel "straight."

We have stretch receptors that tell us when a muscle is stretching or expanding. We also have joint receptors that tell us the relationship of parts to each other. When change occurs they tell us what the movement was and in what direction. When you rigidize joints, as in holding a static posture, you get no information from your joint receptors, like the spindles. With no information it is difficult to make an intelligent plan of action, so we tend to hold on to what we have and it is difficult to break out of the cycle. It is interesting to note that half of all the joint receptors in the body are in the neck. The potential for information in the neck is equal to that in the whole body. It must be important. If your neck is stiff and held in one position you rob yourself of this valuable information.

By not holding on to a stiff and straight posture we are able to receive messages of change and process them. For when the neck muscles are not held, they remain at a slightly stretched resting length (a suspension) which in turn creates a tensional balance throughout the body. F. M. Alexander called this the primary controlling mechanism. Spiritual teachings call it harmony with the universe or oneness. Traditional religious origins call it being close to God.

In other words, if we are not busy pulling ourselves down in one place or another then our bodies are designed to keep us erect, but not held. It is only by letting go that our systems get the information about where we are and the changes that involves. As we let go, the force of gravity, "heaven's force," pushes us toward the earth, while the resultant force of the earth's centrifugal rotation, "earth's force," takes us away from the earth. These two forces, when we allow them, give us our upright status or "straight stature." If we try to pull ourselves up away from gravity by contracting muscles to stand straight, we are creating excess tension that we later have to let go of, and slump down again. The cycle is then endless. Slump down until you realize it or somebody tells you that you are slumping. Then pull yourself up until your muscles get too tired to hold you up and you slump down again.

Practical and workable advice would be to allow the muscles in the neck to be free, which would free the head to come slightly forward and slightly up. As the head frees slightly up, the vertebrae can lengthen and have a bit more space between each one, and then widen, giving more fullness to the ribs and therefore lungs and breath. As the torso has a little bit more space this spirals out through the arms and down through the legs. That little bit of space all over allows heaven's force and earth's force to give us what we want to call good posture.

F. M. Alexander was a rare and remarkable human being. Quoting Marjory Barlow,

74

When Alexander was nearly 80 years old he said to me, 'I never stop working on myself—I dare not.' He knew that the only limits to this kind of development are those which we impose on ourselves.

He continued to teach to within five days of the end, at the age of 86 and then, having refused all drugs which might deprive him of it, he achieved the rare distinction of being present at his own death.[25]

*   *   *

The student learns by daily increment,
The way is gained by daily loss,
loss upon loss until
at last comes rest.
By letting go, it all gets done;
the world is won by those who let it go!
But when you try and try,
the world is then beyond the winning.[26]

—Lao-tzu

3. Movement Related to Lifestyle, Climate and Culture

"When Gulliver stayed in the Lilliputian Isles, he enjoyed himself very much and laughed at the natives' false conception of the world, and at their lack of physical power. But when he landed in the Giant's Country, he had to bewail his own lack of strength, his own ignorance, his false conception of the world, and, at last, his infinite stupidity and ignorance."[1]
—Jonathan Swift

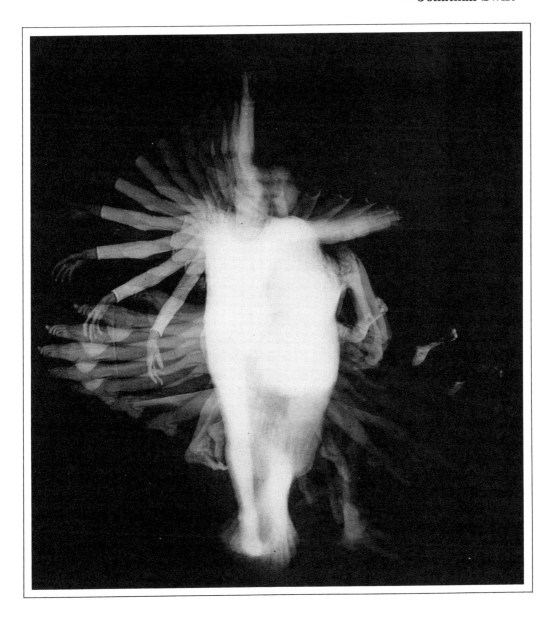

1. Diet and Movement

How does our diet affect the way we move as individuals or in large cultural patterns?
If we look at the world and understand that environment and climate create food,
which turns into energy for thought and action, we can see some general patterns
for movement.

The climate, temperature, terrain, and rainfall as influenced by the action of the
atmosphere and by the celestial motion of the planets, sun, and moon, determine
the kind, quantity and quality of food that grows in a certain area. This food has
received vibration and nourishment from the environment, soil, sun, and rainfall.
If there is a lot of sunshine the plants will be dry. If it rains a lot, they will be wet.
If the field is next to a factory that vibrates all day, that too will influence the crop.
The book and movie, *The Secret Life of Plants* has demonstrated this well.

Traditionally people who live in specific regions will eat the food grown there.
Modern society has changed that to a great extent due to manufacturing and shipping, but many people still eat locally grown food.

After eating, energy is produced and people move through their daily lives. This
movement is influenced by the foods eaten. A very simple example of this would be
the feeling experienced after eating a meal of meat, potatoes, and heavy sauces: you
are full and usually want to sit down and relax for a while. There is a lack of
lightness, spontaneity and desire for movement, whereas after a meal of grains and
vegetables, one tends to feel buoyant, lighter, and active, and when not accustomed
to this style, one is "still hungry."

These characteristics often extend to groups. Members of the same family are often
identified by their similar movement patterns, created from imitation and from the
same dietary habits. On a larger scale this is reflected in the movement tendencies of
society as a whole.

A. General Movement Tendencies

	Cold Weather More yang	Hot Weather More yin
Climate	Cold is actually a yin trait, but produces yang characteristics.	Heat is actually a yang trait, but produces yin characteristics.
Diet	More animal food, salt, and root vegetables.	More sugar, fruit, and vegetable foods (leafy vegetables).
Movement	Closer to the ground, less movement, center-based moving, foot activity, angular shapes, direct moves.	Higher in the air, more movement, peripheral moving, hand activity, flowing shapes, indirect moves.

Illus. 1

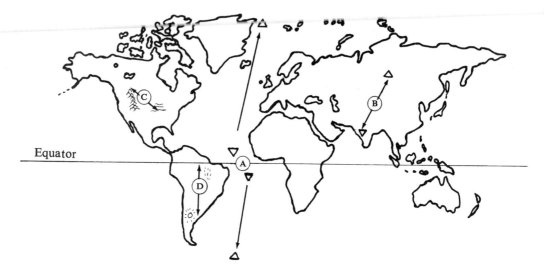

▽ Yin = more expanding energy—more movement
△ Yang = more contracting energy—less movement
    A.   Equator to north and south: yin to yang
    B.   Coastal to inland: yin to yang
    C.   Wide lowland to high, cold mountain: yin to yang
    D.   Hot, wet, rainy climate to cold, dry: yin to yang

In an agrarian-based society, dances were those of fertility, asking for sun or rain, and were followed by dances of thanks to the gods of nature. Then the crops were eaten. When a culture was based on hunting, dances were aggressive, asking for strength and power to kill during the hunt. These also were followed by dances of thanks to the gods for help. Then the killed animals were eaten. Dance naturally grows out of the current cultural consciousness created by food and environment.

Greek society, primarily agriculturally based, gave rise to a dance tradition that was orderly, respectable, and highly developed, even Spartan to the extreme. Later the Roman Empire began to import food from their conquered provinces. Excesses of food and drink in the wealthy class led to wild dances and orgies. This was one way to discharge the excess energy. Areas in which the population eats local food tend to support the same dances over the years. On the other hand, countries which import food have changing dance styles. By looking at climate, movement, and diet in various countries we find some interesting parallels and comparisons.

B.   Cross-cultural Studies

Cross-cultural studies have been done comparing movements of different peoples.

1.   A Yemenite dance was compared to an Indian war dance done by the Thunderbird Indians living in New Jersey. They both had similar steps in space and weight shifts, but their relationship to the ground was different.

The Indians stepped pressing into the ground with strong weight in contrast with the Yemenites, who seemed to touch the ground with lighter weight and rebound into sustainment. Perhaps the Indian diet consisted of more red meat, producing a heavier feeling, while the Yemenite diet consisted of chicken, producing a lighter and flying feeling.

2. Another study was done comparing a North African with a Scandinavian while they were polishing an object, a gourd or bowl.

The North African used curved figure-eight or serpentine moves, flowing shapes, and indirect sweeps over the surface. As she worked, the supporting hand counter-shaped the polishing hand. In a warm climate, the diet is more yin, consisting of vegetable-quality foods.

The Scandinavian used a more linear approach with inward-directed small circles. The supporting hand was still, stabilizing the bowl, exhibiting a more yang quality. The Scandinavian was less smooth and more energized (yang) in contrast to the easy flowing mobility of the African (yin). Again, these movement tendencies are both adaptations to the environment.

3. Opposite movement tendencies can be seen in comparing the Arctic Caribou Eskimo with the tropical Micronesian native.

Arctic Caribou Eskimos take a wide frontal stance. They move so that the whole body moves simultaneously, a mode of action that produces the maximum power needed for spearing animals. The Eskimo moves with straight, linear actions and changes direction with sharp, angular transitions, using space economically because of the ice and cold. His diet consists almost solely of animal-quality food, as little vegetation grows in the ice and cold.

The tropical Micronesian employs a rhythmic up and down motion of pelvis and legs, establishing a pulsating base. This results in a rocking chest motion, flowing segment by segment to outstretched arms, and intricate use of forearms and hands. His motions flow smoothly with curved spatial patterns. His diet is almost solely vegetables, sugar, and fruit.

4. Island people, because they are surrounded by water, demonstrate many similarities. Tropical, hot islands around the world produce strikingly similar body movements.

Examples:

Java—slow movements, swaying to a spiraling rhythmic surge, creating a soothing quality.

Hawaii—using somewhat sinuous body contractions like breaking waves, very flowing.

Philippines—use very flowing arm movements.

Island people from hot climates all eat a diet consisting of tropical fruit, vegetables, and fish, and breathe the warm ocean air.

Cold island people, on the other hand, tend to exhibit less movement, less writhing body movements, and more sudden actions. For example, people from Japan and Ireland maintain straight torsos and bend their arms and legs at the joints. The Irish have more downward energy, as seen in their traditional clog dancing, while the Japanese have a bit more upward energy as seen when they slide across the floor to walk in Noh dance. The diet in both countries consists of grains, root or cold-climate vegetables, and again fish, but here a more dried, salted variety (more yang), and in Ireland, more meat.

C.   General Food Tendencies

General food tendencies correlated to movement are:

1.   *Salt and meat*—heavy, closer to the ground, less movement to no movement. Also explosive or violent movement.

2.   *Fish*—segmented movements. When you eat fish you can see the segmented musculature. This vibration is carried to movement.

3.   *Dairy*—shows heaviness in hips and breast. Excess animal fat tends to collect in unused or stagnating muscles, often obvious around the upper thighs and hips. There are 700 varieties of cheese in France. Is it by coincidence that they developed the cancan dance?

4.   *Grain*—slower, evenly sustained, erect spines, less compulsive desire to dance, less fluctuated movement.

5.   *Vegetables*—lively, solid, but light moves.

6.   *Oil*—fluid, loose, flowing movements.

7.   *Fruit*—lighter, more arms, floating or watery movements.

8.   *Spices*—sudden sharp moves.

9.   *Drugs and chemicals*—strange robot-like, less human, organic movement.

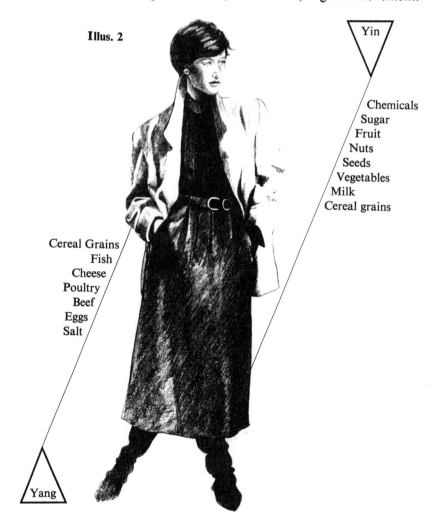

Illus. 2

Yin

Chemicals
Sugar
Fruit
Nuts
Seeds
Vegetables
Milk
Cereal grains

Cereal Grains
Fish
Cheese
Poultry
Beef
Eggs
Salt

Yang

These are very general tendencies, as many other factors also affect our movements, but the ideas may be used to alter our own dance or movement style. If my body is stiff (almost brittle) from too much meat and salt, I can eat more fruit and vegetables to lighten and loosen myself. If I am often pulled down close to the ground, I can eat food that has an upward vibration (leafy greens) to change this. (See Illus. 2.)

D. Examples Reflecting Food and Social Strictures

China, Japan and Korea: all grain-eating cultures where movement is characterized by erect spines. In the martial arts, a wide diagonal stance is assumed with a three dimensional action sphere around the body. Japanese Noh dancers use deep, sustained, slow movements that are precise, direct and generally more yang, moving from the center out (yang to yin). They prefer a natural line and there is no strain for form. They wear masks, show little emotion, and are clothed in tight, stiff, heavy costumes, reflecting a small island with little room to move. They eat a diet of rice, fish, and vegetables.

India: we see more upper body, hand, foot, and head gestures (the yin peripheral), bells, sheer material garments and airy costumes, all more yin, reflecting a warm climate, spicy food, and sugar.

England: court aristocrats danced formally with bulky clothes, stiff corsets and wigs on their heads while eating rich, imported and refined food at banquets. Peasants, still poor and eating dark bread, danced loosely and lively.

Africa: moving to a rhythmic drum beat with whole body involvement. Sugar and tropical fruits are primarily consumed in Africa, a more yin producing, hot climate.

Cuba: the sudden moves of the rumba, a burst of sugar energy.

Burma: back curved, knees bent, faces smiling, grain and vegetable eaters.

Cambodia: delicate and dream-like quality. More southerly; thus, more yin climate and food.

Siam: more action in the dances, more yang climate and diet.

Spain: fandango, flamenco—sudden and sharp, exciting, colorful and intense. Spices, tomatoes, and some animal food in a warm climate.

Germany: methodical, more grounded, little arm or torso movement. Meat and salt, more yang, cold climate.

Russia: low to the ground (yang), foot movement. Much activity and huge jumps in the air, like the effect of a shot of vodka! Less vegetables, more yang, cold climate.

American Indian (Blackfoot):   pure direction up/down, forward/back, not side to side; absence of rounded shapes, intense strength, directness, and suddenness. Yang qualities from a yang lifestyle.

In the Mediterranean Basin folk dances are all similar—lively, colorful, and bouncy. But local variations can be seen—some more sudden due to spices, some more heavy due to salt, oil, and animal fat consumption, and some lighter from fruit and alcohol.

Characteristics of Some Folk Dances

1. *Hungary:* bouncy, energetic, using the hands to clap rhythm on the body.
2. *Brazil:* synthesis of African, European, and native, with the vigor of samba, spiral bodies, bright colors.
3. *Yugoslavia:* heavy, deliberate steps, slow movement with many stops, constant step hop to keep the beat.
4. *Spain:* use castanets, foot stamping, moving hips and swinging arms.
5. *Quebec:* foot tapping, intricate rhythm.
6. *Greece:* the dancing is lively, bouncy, and used to celebrate all occasions.
7. *Armenia:* dancers float effortlessly with gliding steps, light arms, and a lot of repetition, creating a hypnotic effect. The costumes and steps have changed little from Byzantine times.
8. *Mexico:* foot stamping, colored dress, and hats.
9. *Romania:* they use sticks to keep the beat, with a lot of exuberant foot work.
10. *Japan:* folk dances are repetitions of simple motions.

Some movements are designed according to their geographic location. The dance rings of the Blackfoot Indians opens toward the East for the sun; Mexican Cora execute riding dances to the four sacred directions; while the Pawnees of North America paint themselves half red and half black for the dance and turn the red side to the East and the black side to the West. Other dances are designed according to planetary influence. In Southern Brazil, south of the equator, the Cayapo celebrate the day of the new moon, dancing with banana and palm leaves. The Australian Watchandi also celebrate a moon dance. In winter movement is more quiet, whereas in summer it is generally more active. At the time of the full moon activity is higher, and during the new moon the activity level is lower.

All countries that bordered the Mediterranean in ancient times appear to have had a "whirl dance." In Egypt today, the dervishes whirl about constantly in a counter-clockwise direction with arms outstretched. The dancer loses the feeling of body and self and conquers dizziness. The significance is apparently astral, drawing influence from the sun, moon, and revolving stars and planets. It is preserved from a period thousands of years before Islam, probably inherited from Central Asian shamanism. In Hebrew, the word *mahol* is used for women's dances and it derives from the verb meaning "to turn." Perhaps these dances originated in countries that were close to the equator, where the movement of the earth's rotation was strongly felt.

E. Importing Food and Dance

The rise of ballet and the consumption of excess refined sugar have a surprisingly parallel growth. Presented to any traditional culture, ballet would never have been accepted or adopted years ago, but with today's modern diet and way of life, many cultures have a ballet company.

As we read, ballet began in the courts. In France ballet began to really flourish in the eighteenth century. Interestingly, at this same time "middle eighteenth century France moved into the front ranks of the sugar trade."[2] This becomes clear when we know that refined cane sugar comes from a hot, yin-producing climate and grows in tall, thin stalks. The energy created by this plant is upward, graceful in the air, and light, very similar to the motives of ballet dancers. Today almost every financially thriving country whose populace consumes a "modern" diet of imported and refined foods, as well as excess meat and sugar, has a ballet company. "Backward," poverty-stricken countries whose people consume a more traditional diet based on locally grown foods, do not. Ballet is imported like the food in modern countries.

Internationalism is wonderful, but it may prove meaningless to adopt a piece of another culture without fitting it into the whole. For example, there are very few Americans who can perform Spanish dance well. Most do not have the temperament and attitude that make it work. Many dances of one culture do not "look right" on another culture. As the second culture adopts a dance, it can: 1) imitate all the steps and expressions, or 2) change it to suit its lifestyle. Again we need spiral thinking. Because another culture's food or dance is different, we are attracted to it. Yet we want to preserve our own culture. The union of these is change or progress.

There are adaptations in dance as time, society, diet, and way of life change. When Noh was popular in Japan in the 1800s, people ate rice, together with the traditional diet. Now that the Japanese import American food—hamburgers, soft drinks and so on—most young people have little interest in traditional dance or traditional ways. Modern Japanese society has given rise to many avant-garde dance companies.

In the case of ballet, dancers have changed the steps subtly to suit their needs. In the early books of ballet treatise by Carlo Blasis, the arabesque was low and formed a graceful line in proportion to the body's ability to bend.[3] (See Illus. 3). Today the arabesque is taken very high, above 90 degrees, which is a difficult range for most people to accomplish without destroying the integrity in the rest of the body. (See Illus. 4.)

Illus. 3—1820

Illus. 4—1987

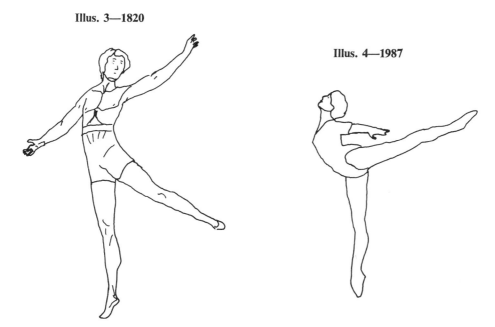

Compare American social dancing of the 1920s to now, and note the accompanying dietary changes. In the twenties, males and females danced together in fun and love and had little processed or chemical food. In 1985, we saw that break dancing was popular among young people. Youths felt trapped and wanted to "break out" of something, but they didn't know what. With head spins and back spins, they accurately chose the spiral to lead them to the answer. But these movements are isolated, robot-like, disjointed, quick, and lacking total body flow patterns. They are usually done to a loud record—staccato, broken-up music—and done one at a time, with little group unity. This dance accurately reflects the mood of young people, most of whom eat a highly chemicalized extreme meat and sugar junk-food diet. This break-dancing society is characterized by the breaking-up of families, and homes with no central hearth, fast food, drugs, crime, and much mental and physical sickness. It is clearly a reflection of our modern, technological way of life.

F. Food and Body Structure

Many dancers are often worried about their weight and want to stay slim, because they do not want to look fat while dancing. The method often chosen is to eat yogurt and/or some cottage cheese variation. This type of dairy food has a tendency to collect in the middle of the body, most notably in the hips. (See Chapter 5, Section 8.) So the area they want to keep slim develops bulges because of what they are doing to stay slim.

We must constantly examine if what we are doing is getting the result that we want. Michio Kushi once said what we don't like will not hurt us but what we *do* like will. We will tend toward excess.

A wiser choice over a yogurt or cheese lunch would be a meal of whole grains and vegetables, and maybe a small piece of fish. The grains slowly release their sugars to give long-term stamina, and vegetables are consumed for vitamins and minerals. This will produce the feeling of lightness desired, as opposed to the heaviness created by animal fat. The slow release of complex carbohydrate (grain) sugars eliminates the "sugar-rush"-to-depression cycle.

We can carry this idea to individual body structure. A person eating a lot of yin food will often grow taller, while a person eating more yang food will be shorter. Examining just one body part—the feet—an excess of yang food creates turned out feet while an excess of yin food creates turned in feet.

Going further we can see specific foods creating movement and thus body types. An obvious example is alcohol. We can recognize the movement patterns of someone who has had too much alcohol (yin). Someone who has eaten a lot of chicken may often have skinny lower legs, just like a chicken, and their movement follows suit. Excess refined sugar is known to produce hyperactive movement, especially in children.

Then we have discharge movements created by excesses, such as snoring—the body trying to discharge excess liquid, or foot tapping—the body's attempt to discharge excess yang energy. Excess talking, singing, and crying are all forms of discharge.

Going back even further, we can examine the reasons for birth defects. A birth defect can always be figured out by yin and yang. Once the cause is determined, a more suitable diet and movement pattern can be used to help the problem. For example, a club foot is caused by excess yang, which may be cold, lack of food, tension, or excess salt and meat. The yang force has held the foot in and not allowed it to grow out. A rehabilitive process would include flowing and outward movements of the foot (not leg), and letting go of whatever it was that held the foot in (inhibition).

2. Diet for Human Movement

"We dig our graves with our own teeth."

—Unknown

A. Similar Patterns in Plant and Human Growth

1. Dahlia (Fig. 1) and comet path (Illus. 5)
2A. Meridian on squash (Fig. 2A) and human (Illus. 6)
2B. Meridian ends on cucumber (Fig. 2B) and on foot (Illus. 7)

Fig. 1

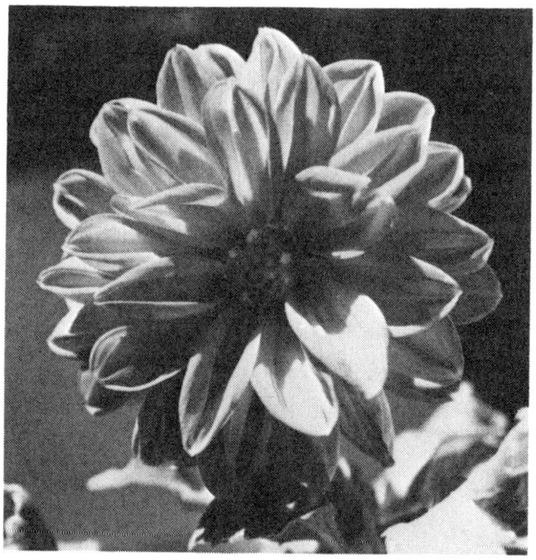

Illus. 5

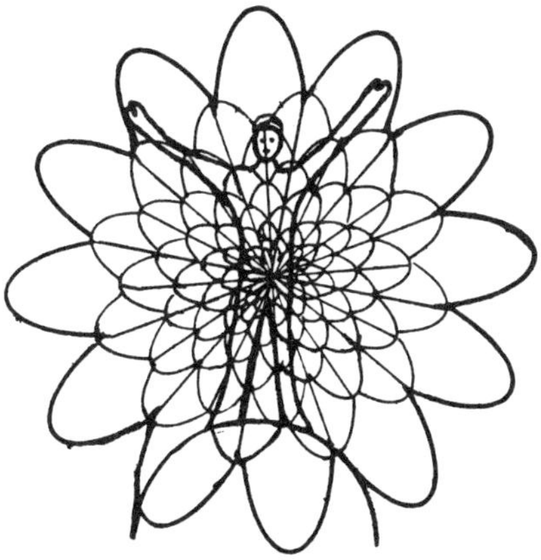

Fig. 2A 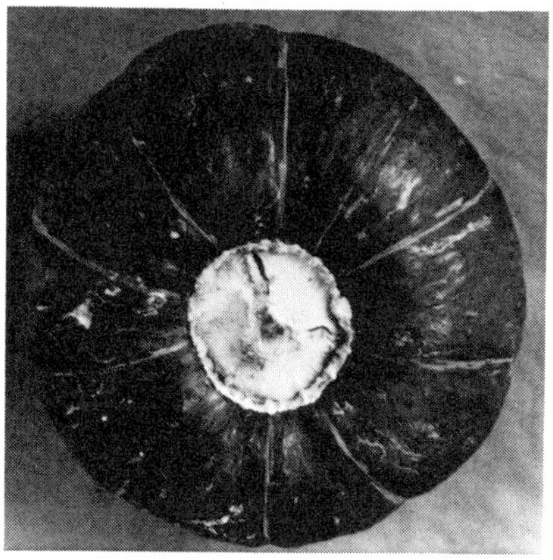　　　**Illus. 6** 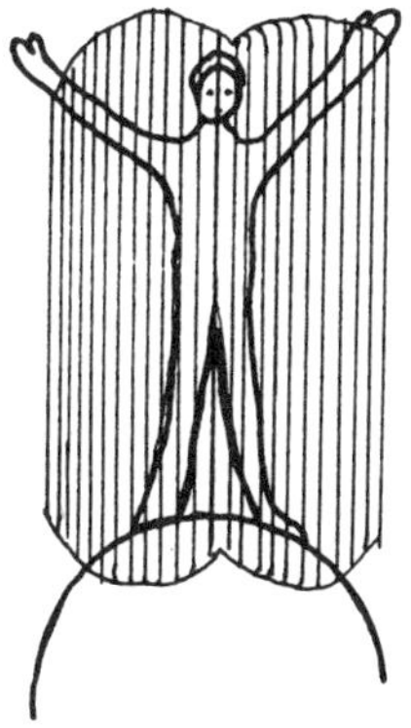　　　**Fig. 2B**

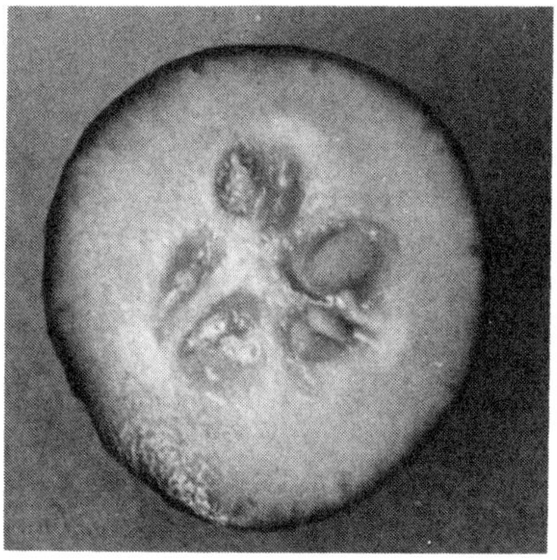

3. Heaven and earth in apple (Fig. 3) and in human (Illus. 8)
4. Spiral in grass (Fig. 4) and in head (Illus. 9)
5. Diagonals in a palm tree (Fig. 5) and in human (Illus. 10)

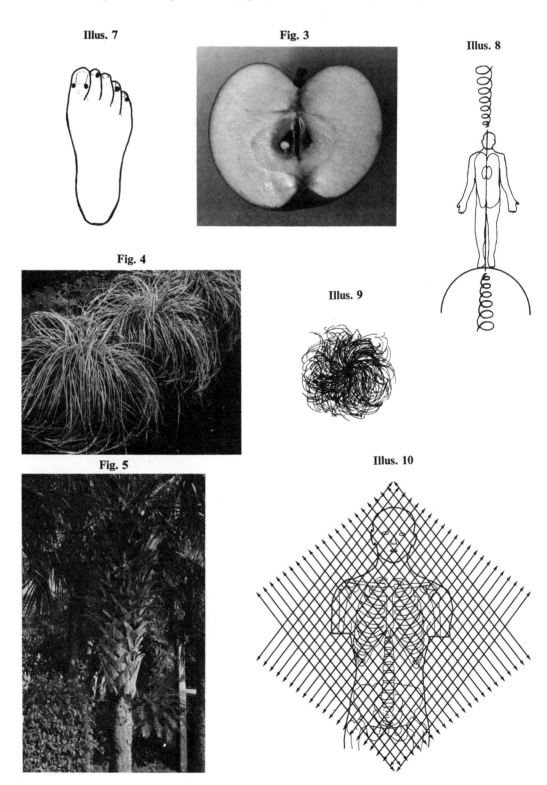

Illus. 7

Fig. 3

Illus. 8

Fig. 4

Illus. 9

Fig. 5

Illus. 10

B. Macrobiotics and Me

As a child I never ate meat. My mother fed it to me but "it would not go down." At that age, it had nothing to do with principles, such as killing animals or the world economy, I simply did not like the taste, texture, smell or anything about it. So I did not eat it.

When I was fifteen years old, I met a man who told me that if I didn't eat meat I should eat whole grain (brown) rice so that my body would receive something nutritious. I came home and discussed it with my parents (my father, a doctor), and we all agreed it was a good idea. So either my mother or I cooked River Brand brown rice every night.

When I was sixteen my friend took me to Michio Kushi's house for dinner. I remember the clean white aprons of the cooks, the Oriental tone, the quiet non-intruding manner, and the strawberry pie that was not sweet.

As a dancer in the early seventies, I wanted my body to work as efficiently as possible for me. As the extras fell away, I became "macrobiotic." The order of elimination seems common:

1. chemicals and drugs
2. meat and sugar
3. chicken and excess of dairy
4. fish and fruit
5. salads and raw foods (vegetables)
6. cooked vegetables (land and sea) and beans
7. whole grains

Naked in the center, I was ready to begin the outward spiritual journey.

Macro (=great) *biotics* (=life) means exactly this. Whatever you do with your life that creates "great life" is macrobiotic. Even if you are healthy, if your direction is toward degeneration, great life is difficult to achieve. Yet even if you are very ill, physically, mentally, or spiritually, and you change your direction toward regeneration, the great life is yours. Eating a diet of primarily whole grain and vegetable-quality food, free of chemicals, can often restore health. Since I have been involved with macrobiotics, I personally have known people to recover from sicknesses ranging from allergies to cancer, and infertility to herpes. This part is relatively simple (but not always easy). A physical law: if you feed the body properly, it will operate properly. Real macrobiotics, however, is more complex: it is acceptance of all without attachment to it, living a free life with no slavery to food, ideas, money, or people, and believing and living that we are all one.

I see it as fullness of being, for the great life leads to a fuller existence on all conceivable levels. Fullness of being is not only the outward expression of physical movement and personality, but also the inward attitude that radiates outward from the core of our very beings. This is "me" only because I have chosen or decided this, and it is manifested in my habits and my association with myself and my environment. I am free to change my attitude, muscular habits, food, and way of life. Some philosophies believe that unhappy people belong in jail, and criminals belong in hospitals. George Ohsawa said that happiness is "endlessly pursuing your infinite dream."

C.   To Begin Health

1.   Eat whole foods grown in your environment so that you are in harmony with nature around you. If this is not possible, eat food grown in your same climatic zone. For example, if you live in a temperate four-season climate, eat food grown in a temperate, four-season climate. Your body will then be suited to weather changes and vibrations that surround you.

Mangoes thrive in a hot climate. Imagine a mango tree in a New England snow storm. It would not last long. It is the same for us if we eat out-of-season food for an extended period of time. I did an experiment with my children. We put an apple and a carrot in the front yard in the fall and watched what happened to them. Then they understood what happens to their bodies by eating either one.

2.   Eat when hungry and drink when thirsty and stop when not quite full—learn to listen. Our senses are unreliable. We eat food that is making us sick and even killing us *and we enjoy it*! We often refuse to give it up even on "doctor's orders." What happened to our "survival instinct" or our intuition? Why do our senses think it is "good?" As we begin to regain our senses with a clearer mind and body, we can then judge for ourselves what is a macrobiotic diet. I may need broccoli today while you may need kale. That big dessert may look good now, but how will I feel tomorrow? I then have a choice: I can eat it and experience the result, or I can refuse it. I know when I am hungry or what is good for me if I am ill. My body will crave what I need to cure my sickness. We are inundated all the time with false advertising and unreliable sensory data, but we do not need to be blindly ruled by them. In many cases it requires a great deal of self awareness and attention to free ourselves from the false patterns that surround us.

Bhagwan Shree Rajneesh explains two kinds of food.[4] The first is called "humming food." Meditate when you are hungry. Close your eyes and feel what your body needs. Perhaps this is the moment of thanks. Eat as much of this as you choose. It will not hurt you, but will satisfy you. The second type is called "beckoning food." You had no desire for it, but you walked past the bakery and it smelled or looked so good that you want some. This will not satisfy you because there is no need in your body for this. But because you are unsatisfied you will eat more of something that there was

Fig. 6

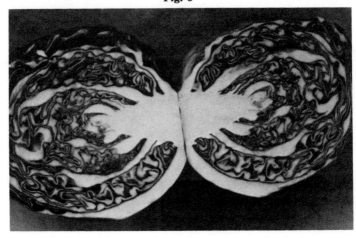

no need for in the first place. Once the first type of eating is fulfilled, the second will disappear. Most people never listen to the first, so the second becomes a problem.

I may crave sugar (yin) which at first has a releasing effect on the body. However, instead of eating sugar I could do a releasing activity such as breathing differently or taking a walk in nature. Or I could substitute the quality. Refined cane sugar, a partial product, can be replaced by eating barley or rice malt (a whole food). For these substitutions, the book *Transitions to a Macrobiotic Diet* is recommended. (See Bibliography.) My body wants to be in harmony with nature because we are ruled by the same force. There is no such thing as going against nature—and surviving—for too long.

If one eats when hungry and stops when full, there would be little problem of excess weight. In continuing to eat we are often searching for something. The body needs vitamins, minerals, and protein as well as universal, spiralic, growing energy (see Fig. 6) to feel satisfied. This is not always supplied by fast, refined foods in a modern diet.

Aveline Kushi tells an amusing story. God gives each of us at birth a certain amount of food. If we eat it all quickly, it is gone, so we die young. But if we eat moderately, the food lasts and we have long life.

D.   What Not to Eat

When we are changing from a standard modern American diet to a standard macrobiotic diet, the order is often similar unless the person is very ill and must change everything immediately.

1.   First, we stop feeding our system any kind of chemical, drug, or synthetic food. Our human bodies are not designed to handle foreign material in any quantity for any length of time. We don't want to resemble hazardous waste sites. Chemicals interfere with our working mechanism. They are not made of spiralic energy and we cannot break them down and eliminate them, whereas anything that grows naturally supports our spiralic nature.

Fig. 7

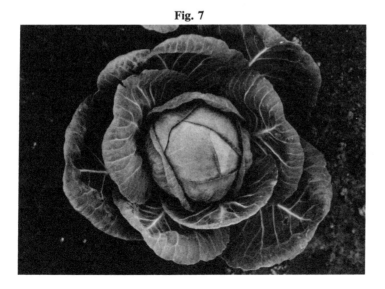

There are many books and magazine articles that explain in depth the harm that chemically-produced foods and drugs create.

2. Meat. The vast acreage of land presently used to raise livestock could feed up to twenty times more people if planted with food crops instead. Not eating excess meat may be understood from a variety of angles. It takes a lot of grazing space to feed one cow. Cows must be fed 21 pounds of protein to produce one pound of protein for humans, whereas the same field planted with grain would feed many more humans with much less time, energy, and effort—in raising, killing, shipping, storing. Biologically we have only four canine teeth (12.5 percent) and 20 grinders (62.5 percent) for grains, and 8 cutters (25 percent). If we eat meat, it should never exceed one-eighth of our daily intake, so that we remain in harmony with the way we are designed. The human intestines are thirty feet long and well suited for the long digestion of grasses. But meat putrifies in such a long system. And finally the simple humane reason: how can you pet a cow at the farm with your children in the afternoon and then go home and eat a steak for dinner? He is too close to us in development. . . . Jesus said: "Blessed is the lion which the man eats and the lion will become man; and cursed is the man whom the lion eats and the man will become lion."[6] If you choose to eat some meat, eat some that is lower in fat or cholesterol and try to find organically raised animals (including chickens) that are not diseased.

3. Excess refined white sugar. "In the 1500s, precious little sugar was to be had unless you were invited to court and somebody gave you a pinch, like someone turning you on to cocaine today."[7] The evils of refined sugar—including causing depression, hyperactivity and many degenerative diseases have taken up volumes. Cane sugar is not so harmful when natives who live where it is grown chew on stalks, husk and all. But when it is refined by removing minerals and fiber, the result is a partial product so your body must supply the minerals that the sugar needs to be properly absorbed. Over a long period of time the depletion of minerals causes great disorder. "Sugar is the unequalled number one murderer in the whole history of humanity,"[8] says George Ohsawa.

In Virginia at the Tidewater Detention Home, Steven J. Shoenthaler performed sugar studies. His findings reported a 45 percent decline in formal disciplinary actions for 24 boys during three months on a sugar-reduced diet.[9] "Today the South American Indians think us civilized people 'crazy' in our inordinate hunger for chocolate, a substance that they use only as a drug."[10] The examples rage on.

4. Dairy. The milk of cows is intended for baby calves. A healthy human mother has more than enough milk to supply her newborn with food. In *Milk: Friend or Fiend*, John Tobe informs us that cows' milk was first given to a human baby in 1793, not since Biblical times, as we all imagined. Cows' milk is rich in protein, calcium, and minerals to support the growth and development of a two-hundred-pound calf. Humans do not need this. When traditional peoples ate dairy food it was before pasteurization, homogenization, and the custom of adding synthetic vitamins and later sugar (to yogurt). They usually fermented their dairy products, thus making them more digestible. The saturated fats and high levels of cholesterol have been proven to lead to ill health when taken in excess.

The genetic trait known as *lactose intolerance* is present in 95 percent of Asians, 70 percent of Blacks, 67 percent of people of European and Mediterranean descent, and 18 percent of North American Caucasians. It means an inability to digest milk sugar. Maybe, just maybe, we are not supposed to digest large quantities of milk sugar. The percentages are also revealing. In the low-percentage countries there is the *belief* that milk is good for you and you must drink it—another example of the body's ability to adapt.

Summary of Foods to Avoid:
- Foods grown out of your climate zone
- All unnatural, artificial, and/or chemically processed foods (instant, canned, or frozen and those with preservatives or stabilizers)
- Commercial red meats and poultry
- Foods containing refined sugar, including commercial crackers, cakes, soft drinks, etc.
- Dairy products, eggs, and animal fats, lard, chicken fat, etc.
- Excesses of stimulants, spices, and yeast
- Vegetables containing irritants or mildly toxic alkaloids that are high in oxalic acid, which inhibits the absorption of calcium: tomatoes, spinach, potatoes, eggplant, and peppers—a more complete list may be gained through the macrobiotic books in the Bibliography
- Refined flour products
- Highly processed foods (soy margarine, wine vinegar)
- Dyed or aromatic teas
- Any iced food or drink (shocks the system)

It is highly recommended not to eat directly before sleeping. During a transitional period, these foods may not be so harmful if taken in small quantities.

E.   What to Eat

"Out of wholeness, emerges wholeness, and wholeness still remains."[11]

1.   In biological development man is the most evolved form of animal, and whole cereal grains are the most evolved form of plants. Many cultures believe that grains are a gift from the gods to humans to sustain life. The growing season for brown rice is approximately nine months. Grains are economical to grow and there is enough for everybody. All traditional cultures used grain as their main food: Europe (oats), Russia (buckwheat), American Indians (corn), Africa (millet), and the Orient (rice). Grains can be stored and kept without spoiling for long periods of time. They are the seed and fruit combined into one.

Whole cereal grains should comprise at least 50 percent of our diet. In the first chapter of Genesis, verse 29, God speaks to Adam. "Behold, I have given you every herb bearing seed which is upon the face of all the earth and every tree, in which is the fruit of a tree yielding seed: to you it shall be for meat."

Whole grains are rich in fiber, B-complex vitamins, vitamin E, and phosphorus. They are composed of complex carbohydrates, proteins, fats, vitamins, and minerals in ideal proportion to the needs of human metabolism. When properly prepared and chewed, they provide stability, stamina, and well-being unequalled by any other food known to man.

Fig. 8A **Fig. 8B**

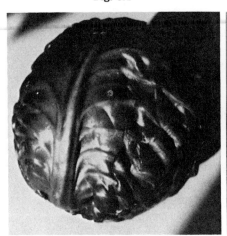 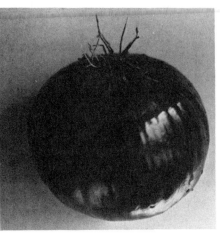

2. Fresh vegetables from the garden delight the appetite as part of any meal. They are rich in vitamins, minerals, and the life force. The colors, tastes, textures, and aromas tell us the nature of the growing season. Leafy greens provide us with upward energy as well as chlorophyll and iron. Root vegetables spiral into the earth; they grow down and impart a secure and stable feeling. Wild (uncultured) vegetables give us the untamed energy of nature. There are many shapes and kinds of vegetables, each giving us different vitamins, minerals, and vibrations. (See Figs. 8A and 8B.)

"There is enough food for everyone's need but not enough for everyone's greed."
—Gandhi

I was once driving in downtown Boston during a walk for hunger. One woman walking was drinking a can of Coca Cola. I wondered if she knew that as long as she continued to drink that, people would be starving. Did she know that fertile soil was used to grow "cash crops," such as sugar cane, instead of growing "subsistence crops" such as grains, beans, and vegetables for the people to eat? There are 5 teaspoons of refined sugar in a can of Coke.

3. Since much of the surface of the earth is covered with water, would it not make sense to eat plant life from the sea? Sea vegetables supply enormous amounts of absorbable minerals. They alkalize the blood, reduce stored fat, and remove poison from the body. They also connect us with the sea, our origin. All traditional people who lived by the water harvested and ate sea vegetables as available food. *Hijiki*, a black, stringy sea vegetable, contains fourteen times more calcium than whole milk. Dulse is 30 times richer in potassium than bananas.

4. Beans are the long lost mate to grains. All traditional cultures have combined the two, somehow knowing that together they provide all the essential amino acids. They provide digestible oils and are very filling when properly cooked. They provide a variety of taste and texture, from *azuki* beans to *tofu* (processed soybeans) to lentil soup.

5. Homemade pickles using no chemicals or sugars are a wonderful source of

fermented enzymes to aid digestion and absorption in the intestines. *Miso* and *tamari* soy sauce are fermented and salted soy products that also provide these valuable enzymes. Pickled plums (*umeboshi*) are very alkaline and are used to relieve any acidic condition and can neutralize harmful microorganisms.

Other recommended foods:
- Seeds and nuts in moderation
- White-meat fish
- Whole-grain products (pastas, noodles, crackers)
- Fruit in season, in moderation (sometimes cooked or dried)
- Grain-based sweeteners
- Non-aromatic teas (*bancha* twig tea)
- Rice vinegar

When choosing your foods try to think about the energy that has created the food. Take, for example, honey: it is made by bees very actively flying around. This energy is found in the food. If you are already overstimulated, this kind of buzzing food energy may not be what you need.

F. Factors to Note in Your Diet

1. The kind of salt—from the land or sea, refined or crude. Refined salt is a partial product with the minerals taken out, so if you eat refined salt your body must supply the minerals to digest and absorb it and thus your body is depleted of its mineral reserves. Unrefined sea salt is recommended for daily use (but not the grey crude type). During the thirteenth and fourteenth centuries, in trans-Saharan trade, salt was traded for an equal weight of gold. Salt-salary was considered to be the ultimate wage, vital to life functions. Salt maintains the blood's alkaline state. Too much or too little salt can lead to problems with the kidneys, circulation, and overall health.
2. The kind of oil—what is it made from? How is it produced or extracted? Unrefined, not cooked oils, are better. Many refined oils use a highly chemicalized process and leave the oil with little taste or nutritional value.

Standard Diet

Every meal should contain 50 percent whole cereal grains, 20 to 30 percent should be vegetables, 10 to 15 percent in volume is cooked beans and sea vegetable, and 5 percent is soup. Fish, fruit, nuts and seeds may be used as needed. Non-aromatic, non-stimulating drinks may be drunk in the quantities needed.

Methods of cooking are very important. We usually do not peel carrots because their vitamins and minerals are just under the skin. When cooking beans which are yin (protein), we always want to add yang (minerals), such as sea vegetable and/or salt. These methods and many more should be learned from a qualified source.

One of the most important factors in the standard diet is chewing each mouthful very well, at least fifty to one hundred times. This is an opportunity to stop and

Fig. 9 — Aveline Kushi cooking

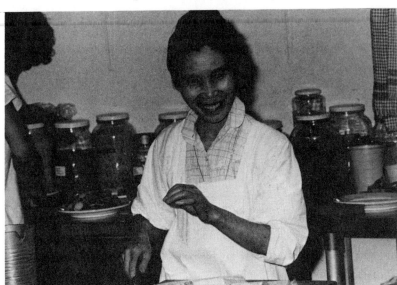

listen. Digestion begins in the mouth and important enzymes are secreted here to break down food so there is less stress on the system further along. The alkaline nature of saliva neutralizes acidic foods. To follow the natural order, chewing is done in a spiral pattern.

It is not only what you do, but how you do it. For the enhancement of the food, we create ambiance while eating. Alone or with friends and family, good cheer, love, and humor make meals pleasant. Taking the time and space to cook and eat is an offering to ourselves. Without these ideas much benefit derived from "good" food can be lost.

If society were healthy, I would end the book here. With a healthy balanced life most sicknesses would be cured in time. But today we must use additional approaches because society is getting so sick so fast. In 1985 one million Americans were estimated to carry the AIDS virus. That figure is predicted to double every year, so in ten years the whole population of the United States would have had some form of contact with the disease.

There are a few humans who have understood an enlightened way of life without a "macrobiotic" diet (based on whole cereal grains), but they soon became sick and could not continue teaching. Yes, they were smart and had understanding but they could not teach their students how to become like them. Their students can be little more than parrots using only their words or movements. However, dietary adjustment changes the makeup and quality of the blood. The blood rich with iron feeds the brain and acts as a magnet to change the whole picture from deep inside, giving us direction and confidence to steer our lives.

3. Recommendations for Daily Healthy Life

Look at daily life. If you don't know what you're doing, you can't do what you want.

We wake up in the morning—
With the sun, or have we overslept and are late for work or school?
Can we use our conscious minds to wake up at a decided time, or do we need an alarm clock?
Was the sleep peaceful?
Is my body tight in any special place?
Any dreams that night?
Do I have a heavy feeling from the night before, attaching myself to it, or am I refreshed and ready to start a new day?

Get up and start to move—
Do I smile at people on the way to the bathroom?
Brush my teeth: how much tension do I use to hold that half-ounce toothbrush?
Do my bowels move smoothly or do I have constipation or diarrhea?
If I was up last night later than my body could handle or ate too much before sleeping, I find it hard to get going, so I have a cup of coffee.
Is my behavior spontaneous or compulsive?
Then we begin to cook breakfast:
Is my kitchen orderly?
Do I try to keep a calm and peaceful mind while I cook?
My thoughts manifest in my body, and through my hands the vibration goes into the food.
If my shoulders are tense while cutting vegetables, that tension or anxiety carries to the finished meal that my family eats.
I cannot wonder why the children are fussy.

In my body—
When I stand, do I lean into one hip?
When I sit, do I cross the same leg all the time?
Do I always step forward on the same foot?
Do I always carry a package with the same arm?
How can I wonder why my body is held rigidly and my thinking is narrow?
When I am tired, I don't sleep.
When I am thirsty, I don't drink.
When I have to go to the bathroom, I hold it in because I am doing something.
When I have pain, I try to ignore it.
When I am not hungry, I eat.
When I am full, I do not stop because it looks or smells so good.
When I eat, I don't chew, I gulp my food down.
When I work, I don't breathe.

Where is health among all these?
Why don't we listen to body signals and messages?

In modern society our senses are perverted at an early age. Often babies are
delivered at the doctor's convenience, not when the child is ready. We are forced to
eat what our body wants to reject, because it is "good for us." If you don't like milk,
your mother puts chocolate syrup in it to get you to drink it. Then you have direct
harm from the sugar, plus you are a slave to the habit. We are often made to sleep
when it is convenient, not when we are tired. In school you eat at the appointed time,
not when you are hungry. As these and more add up, it becomes difficult to differentiate between a natural desire and a desire to please others.

If I choose to take responsibility for my life and actions I can change any of these
things and set my life in the direction I want by observation or listening to the clues
around me. If I am hungry, I eat; if I am tired, I sleep. Through this, I realize and
continue my life dream.

Life is meant to be a dance. We move freely from one aspect to the next. After
understanding misperceptions of food and thought, other aspects making our daily
lives more harmonious are:

1. *Having contact with Nature daily.*   When we have plants, exposed wood and
many windows at home, in the dance studio, or work place, we are surrounded by
calmness, inspiration and a deep stillness. On the other hand, we should not have too
many (of course, there will be some) electrical or technological buzzings around us,
such as fluorescent lights or microwave ovens. We can balance these by watching and
learning from the seasons, the plants, clouds, skies, mountains, and oceans.

2. *Wearing natural fiber clothing, cotton or others, not synthetics, especially next to
the skin.*   I remember the days I was either dancing, teaching, or rehearsing ten hours
a day in nylon leotards and tights. They were so uncomfortable to put on. But once
on I soon forgot. We are such adaptable creatures. But when I took them off . . .
aahh! What a relief. It is funny because as dancers we want ourselves to extend out
but synthetic material does not fully transmit electromagnetic energy, nor allow the
body to breathe. Tight elastic waists or bands on clothes block circulation. A body
scrub with a hot damp towel increases circulation. Shoes that are not flexible do not
allow all the muscles in the feet to work. Tight pants look fashionable and sexy, but
they do not always allow us to bend at the hip sockets properly.

3. *Focusing on mental and spiritual thoughts.*   "The rigor with which we inculcate
the rigidness of human nature is the main source of our misery."[12] We must examine
the way we think. Unreliable senses combined with inappropriate diet give the human
being the idea of self-destruction. No other animal has this idea. If an animal is
hungry he eats. Animals don't eat over anxiety attacks or sneak food, and they don't
diet for being overweight. In mating, they don't seek out meaningful relationships
and from what I know, they don't divorce. Spirit strives for life, to create and continue the spiral.

The ideas of original sin and man being cursed or damned from the start is only
a reflection of the misuse of the human organism. In the ancient Japanese prayer
O-Harai, it is explained that one need only stop and self-reflect (observation) and
recognize (awareness) one's behavior (admit), and without the guilt and the conse-
quent muscle tension, allow one's self to exist more in harmony with the forces of

heaven and earth and infinity. These self-destructive, depressive tendencies can be overcome.

What sin could be so long lasting that man is cursed from birth? Man's law is always relative, taken in context: kill a man on the street, go to jail, kill a man in battle, become a hero. According to natural law, eating excess ice cream or chemicals is a violation. It goes against the natural order and upsets balance. In this light there are many criminals walking the streets. There is no built-in punishment for "sin" except for the fact that we must live with the results of our actions. We misuse our-selves=sin. We must live with the pain=punishment.

As we stop the separation from the wholeness and listen, our habits change. We gradually let go of anger, jealousy, and hatred. This is not through mind manipulation or me convincing you what is good.

Our mental training must then foster pleasant thoughts in loving and supportive environments. If grains are the gift from the gods, perhaps humor is the gift from the goddesses. Laughter has been used through the ages for healing and releasing. Masahiro Oki, a Japanese yoga teacher, used to say, "When a baby is sick, tickle him and he will get better." A smile brings the soft palate back and up, which allows the head to come forward and up.

Again to quote Michio Kushi, "What we do not like will not hurt us, but what we like will hurt us." Because we are attached to what we like, we may experience the excesses of that liking. If food, we will eat too much of it. If it is a body position, we will use some muscles too much and others not enough. What we hold on to may be called our attachment, and what we exclude as a result of it may be called our arrogance. Our arrogance may be said to be anything that we don't like, or choose to ignore. This prevents us from being aware that we are part of a whole, a large universal oneness. Often the sequences or ways of thinking or eating that we feel least like doing are the ones that we need the most.

We must give thanks (prayer) to everyone and everything. (See Fig. 10.) For we all

Fig. 10.

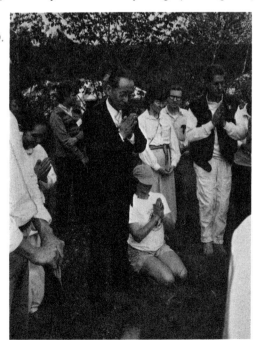

came from one and are all here to balance each other as a part of that one. We give gratitude to parents and ancestors, friends and enemies, good times and bad. We give thanks daily to Nature for our food. We plant one grain and reap ten thousand. We have faith. Gradually as our delusions are fading and our senses become uncovered, our deep intuition sets us on the path. If there is true submission, there is no holding to an attitude or position and the reflexes can respond to the information dictated by the nervous system, which is constantly trying to maintain its dynamic equilibrium.

4. *Being aware of motion in daily life.* There is no way to be here now if you are goal-oriented. The self is to be in the present moment, not reacting to the last moment or daydreaming about the next. Begin from where you are, not where you would like to be. If your mind is busy figuring out another moment in time, you cannot fully be present in this moment in time. One would like to experience this moment with no dialogue or evaluation of it. Carried into movement, when you sit in a chair you do not want to fall back into it and let the chair catch you. If you do, you have lost the moment by moment process, and you have put the muscles in a state of the startle pattern. They feel you falling but they do not know that the chair is there. So they grab as a balance reaction. Rather, moment by moment you want to stay over your support—your feet—and bend at the major joints (ankles, knees and hips), keeping your neck free, not pulled or held in any position. Then you can sit with an educated, present being. As you sit, heaven's force or gravity will assist you. As you stand, earth's force coming up will assist you. If you don't interfere, in both cases. (See Fig. 11.)

The same applies to walking. Give credit to your upright stature by allowing all the muscles to extend to their lengthened resting length and move from the joints. One teacher said that most walking looks like an "arrested fall" and not a movement forward in space. (See Chapter 5, Section 3.)

Fig. 11

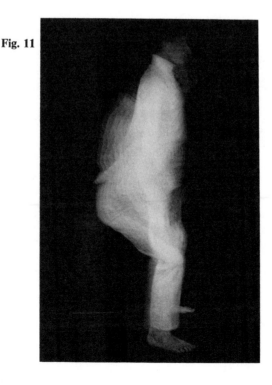

4. Macrobiotics and the Alexander Technique

"Give up control and gain command."

—David Gorman

In the plant kingdom when we examine the process of growth, we begin with a seed and plant it in the soil. With sunlight, air and water the seed splits open and begins to grow. Roots are sent down and a stem grows up. Out from the stem comes branches, twigs, leaves, and finally the flower—the fruit and seed, all coming up from below (Illus. 11).

Illus. 11   **Illus. 12**

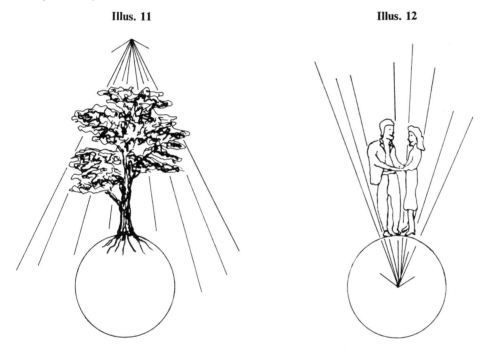

In human growth, a seed planted in water and fed with nutrients, grows to a human form. But in this case the branches grow inward, not outward, as in plants. These are the meridians, veins, arteries, and capillaries, all getting smaller as they go inward to individual cells. In humans, the flower, fruit (baby) and seed come out from below, the lower body, the opposite direction from plant life. (See Illus. 12.) When we understand human form in this way, we can begin to understand some Alexander Technique teachers who say that the body is a large suspension system hung from the head, or as Michio Kushi says, we are "hung from heaven."

This may be an unusual idea to most of us. Because of our physically and materially oriented society we think of ourselves as coming only from the earth. As we have been conditioned to believe that cows' milk is important to a child's growth, we have also been raised to believe that gravity is a force that pushes us down. We must pull up against it in order not to fall. Pull yourself together!

The body is often pictured as a pile of blocks, stacked on top of each other, so we think our muscles are something like pulleys that pull these blocks or bones around. This may be fine for a Walt Disney cartoon but it has no resemblance at all to human life or function. No matter how well you may align yourself, there is no way that your bones will stack up to balance by themselves.

Take one look at a skeleton, especially in the torso. There is built-in imbalance so we can create dynamic (non-static) equilibrium. In addition to gravity, the upward force created as the earth rotates, manifests as a whole system of muscles responding to this energy called the anti-gravity muscles, or extensors. They take you away from gravity. If we allow our anti-gravity muscular system to function then we do not have to pull up, thus eliminating tense muscles and compressed bones and organs. We can be aware of our suspended nature and allow the earth to support us.

From a structural point of view, during the embryonic period the navel functioned as the center of the entire body, receiving food. After birth the center shifted to the head (mouth) and neck region. From here upper and lower body extensions have developed, the head as the upper sphere, the body the lower. The third eye area is the center of the head affecting the nervous system. And the hara, or *tanden*, is the center of the torso affecting the digestive system. Accordingly these two correlate well with each other. In Oriental diagnosis, one may detect the condition of the torso (its internal organs, etc) by looking at the head (the face, its lines, etc.).

As we see the primary importance of the activities centered around the head and neck region, a universal view emerges. In Illustration 13,[13] A is the earth; B the solar wind; C is the centrifugal force generated by the rotation of the earth; D is centripetal force coming from peripheral space toward the center of the solar system. The earth rotates, generating electromagnetic orbits formed by B and D colliding and they in turn form the human likeness of plasmic energy. From this picture it is very clear that whatever goes on in the A area (corresponding to the neck region) greatly influences the entire body. The neck region is the center between two different, equal and corresponding parts.

Mechanically this can be explained by the dynamic imbalance built into our system. When the neck muscles are freed, our head falls slightly forward. Our muscular design includes the stretch reflex. When a muscle is stretched or expanded, another part of the muscle contracts—a safety mechanism to keep us from coming apart. So when the neck and spinal muscles stretch for the head to fall forward, they also contract, each muscle on top lifting the vertebrae below. This produces the feeling of suspension from above. This is something we cannot do, but must allow.

When we allow ourselves to be in this state, the forces of heaven and earth are able to flow smoothly throughout the body, thus connecting us to our infinite origin. Then we do whatever we do more fully present in the moment and our thoughts and actions are not based on past or future determinants.

Another part of this physical reality explaining the uniqueness of the mouth and neck area is the uvula. "There is another organic system composed of cerebral substance, nerves, muscles, and cartilages, which, to the same degree as the hand has determined the superiority of man over all living beings. It consists of the tongue and the larynx and their nervous apparatus."[14] As we have seen, there is a channel or path of energy through the center of the body containing the chakras or energy centers. Energetically it is an unbroken channel except for one spot. Behind the mouth is a separation where the *uvula*, a small piece of flesh, hangs down. Because of the

Illus. 13

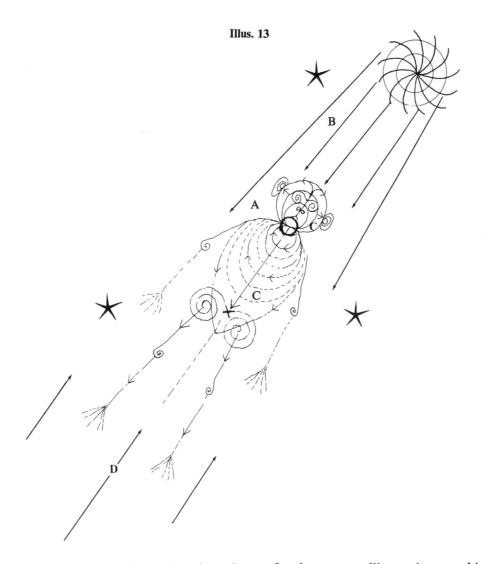

break, this area is our free will and our key to freedom, controlling eating, speaking, breathing and the angle of the head. Macrobiotics emphasizes the front part through the importance of eating, while the Alexander Technique emphasizes the back part through the importance of the state of tonus in the back neck muscles. Front and back of the same area. Any chronic contractions in the neck muscles upset the dynamic balance of the head to torso relationship, and consequently the entire body.

Both the Alexander Technique and the macrobiotic way are a process of education, not a therapy where somebody does something to you or for you. Each of us can be our own master, we need not be slaves to anyone, neither medical professionals nor the media.

In the beginning we need guidance by qualified instructors because there is much erroneous education and our senses are faulty. F. M. Alexander said, "Many adults have a debauched sense of taste because of eating too much sugar-sweetened food in childhood."[15] With inaccurate senses it is difficult to know the correct path. If we have cancer we blindly run to a doctor (but he himself may have cancer). If we have excess muscle tension we go to a chiropractor whose body may also be full of excess tension. Can they possibly help us? A therapist may be able to help others cure symptoms, but a master can help himself as well as help others.

Let us look at the issue of back pain. In our society standing up straight means that the stomach is held in. Therefore, many people do "sit-ups" in order to have a flat stomach. In doing so we are contracting the vertical abdominals which attach to the lower ribs at the top and to the pelvis at the bottom. When a muscle contracts, both ends pull toward the middle. In the case of "sit-ups" we are practicing bringing the ribs closer to the pelvis. In order to stand up "straight" we must pull that front-ward contraction (bending over forward) back up, usually by contracting the lower back. This, of course, creates excess tension in the lower back, because it is always holding you up. The result is pain. Now you go to get some medical help and they will tell you to do "sit-ups" to strengthen your stomach!

There is so much mis-education about how the body is designed to function.

How do we free ourselves from habits? A qualified Alexander teacher or a mirror can help you to develop your kinesthetic sense. You will learn to detect your habitual pattern of holding. Using the means explained, you can allow the primary controlling mechanism to function. Diet can also provide helping or hindering factors. If you are consuming a diet high in animal fat (meat, poultry, eggs and dairy food) then many physical blockages are created, and it is difficult for energy and circulation to proceed smoothly. For example, studies have proven the link between high fat diets and heart disease. In this case, the arteries are actually clogged, hindering the flow of blood and energy throughout the body. If you are consuming sugar, chemicals, and drugs, your mind is unable to focus clearly, hindering your conscious thoughts of freeing the neck area. Studies in this case have linked sugar-coated diets to hyper-activity and learning disabilities in school children. With these constant physical interruptions, productive change is difficult. On the other hand, if you are eating a whole grains-based diet, including vegetables, beans, sea vegetables, and supple-mental fish and fruit, and chewing well, your system is given substance that the body can digest, absorb, and distribute comfortably. The body then functions in a more harmonious state, creating a sense of lightness and well being.

Although F. M. Alexander did not follow the standard macrobiotic diet, his well cultivated ability to listen to his body led him to pay particular attention to quantity, quality, and manner of eating, preferring whole (brown) products to refined (white), and avoiding chemicals, iced foods, and overeating.

As you begin to listen to your body (self-reflection) and your senses are more aware, you will find it is difficult to overeat or eat a lot of heavy or chemicalized food. You will get a message from your body. Now enters that great gift bestowed only to mankind—freedom of choice. You may decide as you hear the signal, yes, I want to eat it, or no, I do not want to eat it. But you must realize that you do not have to be a slave to your reactive habits. Most of us operate on automatic pilot and never notice that conscious control is available.

In this example you may replace the food with any behavior response pattern (emotional or practical, for instance). You have the freedom to react habitually or to free your head and neck and allow yourself to be in the universal flow and proceed from there. Again, the word "allow" is so important. It is not something that we can do. The most we can do is to get out of our own way constantly. The intelligence for healing is built in. One example, cortisone is produced in the adrenal cortex and is

Illus. 14

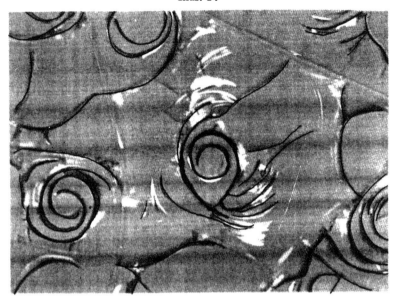

secreted when the body is exposed to stress or strain. Illustration 14 is a drawing of a cortisone hormone crystal magnified 1,000 times.[16] Spiral energy is distributed to restore balance quickly. Many other hormone crystals are angular in shape.

With an all encompassing view and good diet, our day-to-day attachments must melt into the spiral of life. Small issues that we tend to get hung up with create excess tension, but they are very small in the large universe. And this tension prevents us from fully being part of this universal energy which allows us to live more freely.

We all have historical and recent patterns of eating which have influenced our behavior. Once the diet is changed, how quickly does the muscular system of use respond, and to what depth? My personal belief is that the Standard Macrobiotic Diet and way of life will balance all systems in generations to come. The Alexander Technique makes available to us, through the kinesthetic sense, the information necessary to consciously change this pattern of psychophysical use quickly.

For example, you have a lung problem—*functional* (the lung is not functioning properly). Along with this you stand holding one shoulder higher than the other—*structural* (your structure is changed). As you change your diet the function improves but if you are constantly holding that shoulder up and you do not know it, then the function of the lung will be hindered in some way. Use affects function. I think here we can also turn it around and assume that if you correct your shoulder and do not correct your diet, then a deep cure is also difficult. Function affects use.

As we saw earlier, there is a myth in our society that there is a correct "posture" or position. There exists only a more coordinated relationship of the parts. This may be equated to the search for the perfect macrobiotic diet. Again, the principles and relationships are there but we must put the pieces together according to the changes in season, climate, and condition. We are influenced by many changes that take place from moment to moment. We want to deal with reality, not concepts, images, or illusions. We do not imagine the body to be something it is not—like a cloud floating. Neither are we an intellectual theory nor the same as a studied laboratory animal. We must perceive what we are and proceed from there. Practical day-to-day eating, thinking and use determine our relationships.

The mini-version of this book may be: (1) allow your neck to be free; (2) allow your head to come forward and up; (3) allow your back to lengthen and widen; and (4) eat brown rice.

When there is trouble in the body it is never in one place. The whole being is troubled, yet the symptom may show up in a certain part of the body, such as an eye, an organ, limb, etc. If in the eye, we go to an optometrist to seek medical advice, or to an alternative practitioner for the Bates method—but both are treating the symptoms and not addressing the total problem of misuse in food, body, mind, and spirit. We must consider the union of the whole, remembering that the whole is greater than the sum of its parts. Whole food=whole body and whole body=whole food. To evolve is to proceed forward. Because whole grains are the most evolved biological food, they support the forward and up direction of man.

The same is true in society. It is not one person who is sick and separate from the whole: we exist in relationship to the whole. Modern society is based on the startle pattern and a fast-food, highly processed diet. It is not working. Humans are not eating human food. There are no meals. Meals mean grain dishes. Many humans are sick and degenerating. Their movements are hunched over, tense, and inflexible. Chronic sickness and pill taking is accepted as the natural way.

People have lost the lightness and delicacy of human movement. Nearly everyone lives in a state of the startle pattern with fear, distrust and defense ruling and governing ourselves and our systems (insurance, police, and so on). As a result, there is war in every domain, from fighting bacteria to nuclear war. It is just not working. The time for change is now. We cannot wait for a savior (who *will* come). The change begins with you and me in every moment.

There are many popular techniques to learn to do this and train to do that in a new way, and through them changes do take place. One idea that distinguishes the Alexander Technique from them is that you are unlearning and allowing the reflexes to function. This to me is trust cultivated not in ourselves to rule ourselves, but a calling of our deeper nature to sincerely appreciate the natural order of creation. In macrobiotics as well, we are unlearning that we need dairy foods to grow strong, a candy bar for energy, or drugs for every ailment. Instead we eat the foods most biologically suited for human consumption and we live in harmony with the environment. Then, naturally, reflexes take over to create a comprehensive way of life for humanity. Both the Alexander Technique and the macrobiotic way of life provide a means to live by, not an end in themselves.

4. Contemporary Movement Schools

"In America by 1945, in the Journal of the America Medical Association, D. G. Hanson and other medical practitioners recognized the evidence of an intimate relationship between body mechanics and health in preventing disease."
—Raymond Dart

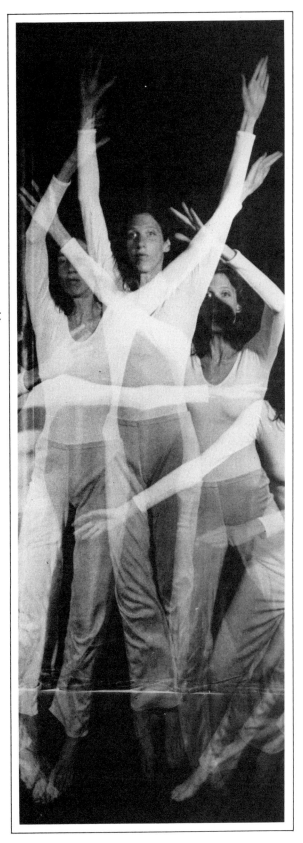

There are a few movement educators whose lifetime study in the field has contributed innovative ideas and methods of understanding the body, energy, human effort, and reaction.

No sense trying to make it look right the wrong way.

—Frances Cott

1. Technical Dance Analysis — Frances Cott

Technical Dance Analysis (TDA) was created and is taught by Frances Cott. Miss Cott started dancing at age three and has continued to dance and teach since. When she was eighteen she met a ballet mistress who was to change the course of her life. Dot Duvall retrained Frances Cott in the Cecchetti method of ballet, as its originator had intended. This method of ballet created by Enrico Cecchetti in Italy emphasizes the natural flow and internal process of the body, not an end pose as is often the case today.

Miss Cott has used this training as a base for her system and has added to it her contact with Wilhelm Reich's orgone energy studies, many styles of dance and movement, and her teaching experience of more than thirty years with students of all ages.

I worked side by side with Miss Cott for seven years, studying with her and teaching at her school in New York. When I moved to Boston I taught her method in dancing studios and movement centers and saw great benefits reaped.

It is a method controlled by the self and not the reflexes. This makes it more mechanical but it is the most efficient and accurate mechanical system I have seen available. It is especially valuable to dancers or persons who actively use their bodies. It allows people to change enough through physical workings of their musculature to develop mental and spiritual understanding. Again, the principles of motion are based on the spirals. The spirals support movement. All ballet positions and steps, when properly executed, are in accord with the spiralic design of musculature, and support a healthy body.

I have presented TDA the way I see it and have added to it any information I feel relevant.

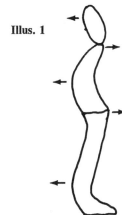

Illus. 1

Most humans today have what is called a zig-zag in the body looking something like this or a variation of it. (See Illus. 1.)

These next few pages suggest where our parts would be if we were not busy *pulling* ourselves out of place. Inefficient movement patterns may come from a variety of sources, including imitation, food, sickness, or emotional or enrivonmental conditions.

Beginning with the feet, let us see the most advantageous set-up from a mechanical point of view.

108

Feet

The basic position for a parallel position:

Flex the foot. See two tendons at the ankle bone and an indent between the two (Fig. 1). Draw a line from the indent to the middle toe. Make those lines parallel on both feet.

Look at the foot from the back (use a mirror). The ankle bone should not be rolled in (Fig. 2). If it is (Fig. 3), keep the front of the foot where it is and rotate just the heel bone forward (toward the center of the body). The whole calf should rotate as you rotate the heel.

Fig. 1

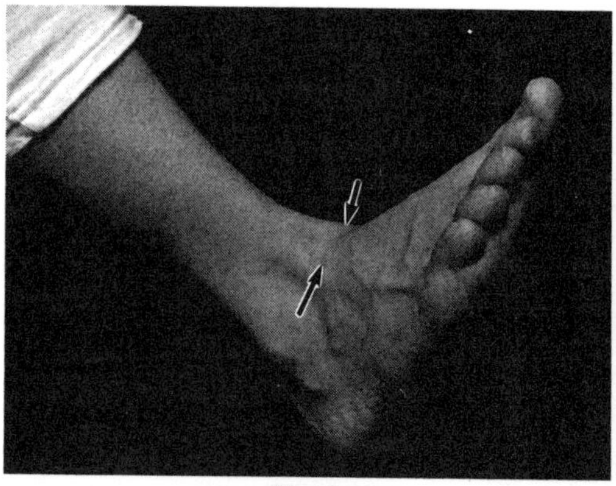

Fig. 2

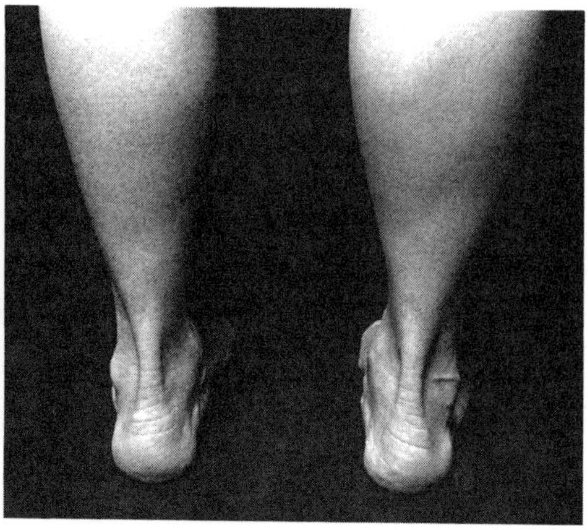

Fig. 3

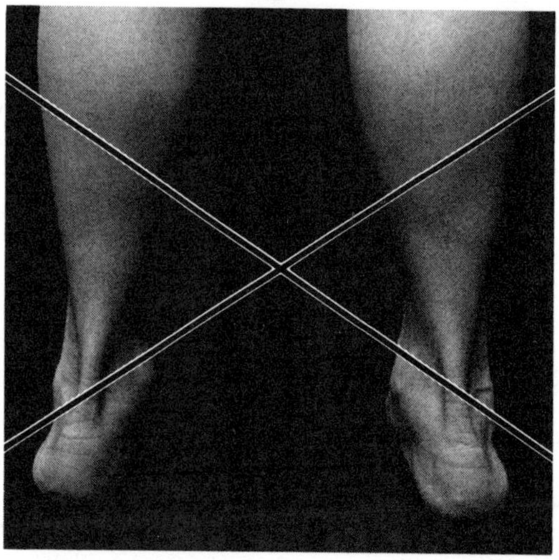

Fig. 4

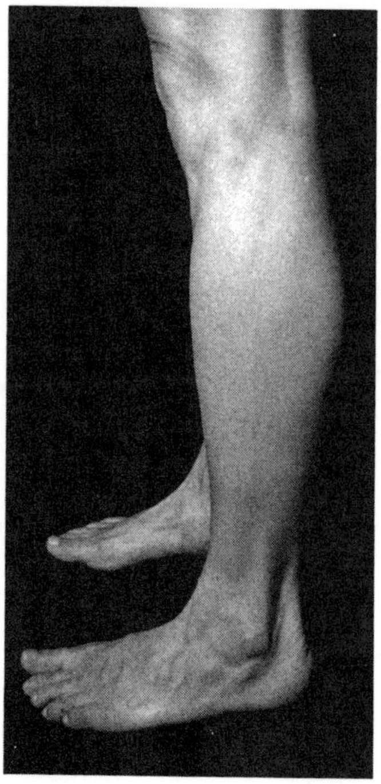

Calf and Shin

The lower leg wants to stand perpendicular to the floor (Fig. 4) (not dropped back).

There is a slight push forward on the shin bone. When you bend the knee the thigh bone often slips down slightly over the lower leg bones. As you straighten, the thigh bone should slip back up into place. Unfortunately it does not always. Along with other factors (twists and bad diet, or others), this causes a lot of knee problems in athletes and dancers.

To counteract this problem:
Pretend you have a knee in the middle of your shin bone. Any time you bend your leg, bend that pretend knee first. It provides more support for the thigh bone. This prepares the way and allows the calf to let go enough to free the knee forward and away as in Alexander's direction.

Knee

The knee is not one specific bone or muscle. It is a space with a cap. One must talk about the calf or thigh to effectively explain or change the knee.

Thigh and Pelvis

In order for maximum rotation of the femur in the hip socket, the bottom of the pelvis must come forward and the pelvic crests must be lifted up and back. This is referred to as rocking the pelvis. It means not only verticalizing the pelvis but also lifting it back and up on top of the thighs (Fig. 5). The common term "tuck under"

Fig. 5   Fig. 6

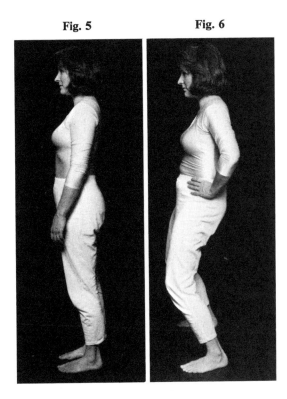

tries to verticalize the pelvis but because there is no lift involved, it serves only to jam the buttocks in behind the thighs, allowing no room for rotation in the hip joint, and building bigger buttocks and thigh muscles (Fig. 6).

Rocking pelvis versus tuck under: pelvis up over thighs versus pelvis pushed in behind thighs.

Process:

Lie on your back. Put your feet on the floor. Relax and breathe. Breathe in and at the end of the out breath tip the bottom of the pelvis up and the top of the pelvis back and up. This is the beginning of rocking your pelvis. Rocking the pelvis prepares one to free the hips back and up as in the Alexander directions.

Shoulders and Upper Body

The body is a set of diagonal pulls, used to accent appropriate lines, especially in ballet (Illus. 2). Do not hold your shoulders. *Breathe* into the upper chest and allow it to widen. Breathe in so that your ribs expand like an accordian. Make them wider. As the upper torso is filled with air, the head is lightly poised on top. Arm movements come from the torso. The forces of heaven and earth meet and spiral out to communicate.

Illus. 2

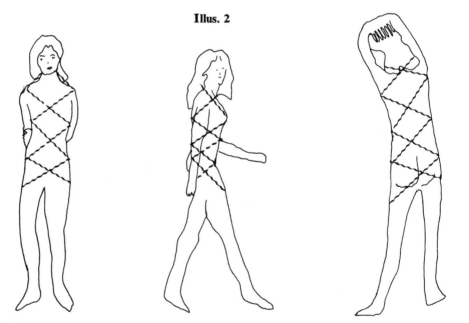

This next sequence uses straps to stabilize and move bones and muscles. They seem unusual but the cures are only the result of the sicknesses that we have created. If we had not created such sickness we would not need to create such a cure.

We all have a way of using our muscles that contracts them in a certain pattern. If we decide we want our muscles to work another way, we may try to change by contracting another set of muscles. In this manner we usually jam one set of muscles against another. Instead, we first must *stop* doing the old pattern. And then have some help to find the new. Either someone's hands, thoughts, or straps are used to change relationships and to redirect energy. Then by ourselves we can direct the new.

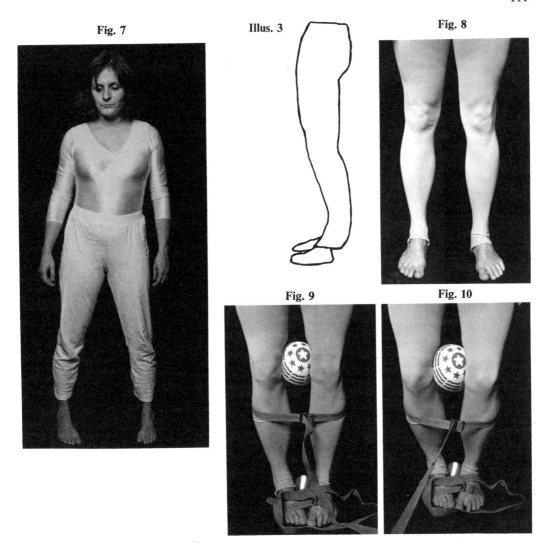

Fig. 7

Illus. 3

Fig. 8

Fig. 9

Fig. 10

The straps hold muscles and bones in a more functional relationship to each other. They are training and developing tools.

Hyperextension is any misalignment of the calf and thigh. One example is a locked knee (Fig. 7) (Illus. 3). Often the ligaments are overstretched and the muscles are short and tight. They can't coordinate to be lined on top of each other so they snap back to hyperextension. The parallel strap process may be used for any problem concerning the relationship of the thigh and lower leg.

Parallel Strap Process:
1.   Stand up (Fig. 8).
2.   Put straps around the metatarsal arches to hold the toes together. Put a spacer between the heels. The spacer can be a small rubber ball. Put another spacer between the top part of the knees so that the bottom (calf) part can move in. Put straps around calves, and pull forward. (Put straps where they lean out the most on the calf.) (Fig. 9)
3.   Bend and straighten in this position (Fig. 10). Read "How to Unfold Leg."

Fig. 11

Fig. 12

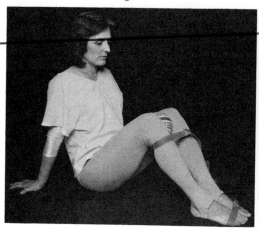

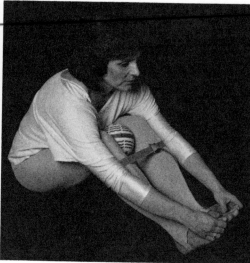

Fig. 13

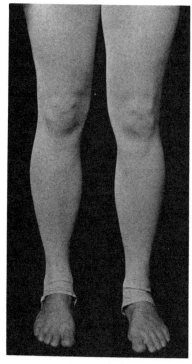

4.   Bend top body over and put your hands on the floor and your back against the wall. Start with hips over heels. KEEP HEELS ON FLOOR. Stick buttocks back and up to straighten. DO NOT PULL CALVES BACK! The knee joint wants more space. Breathe. Top calf should not jam back. Thigh should unfold. Calf stays forward.

5.   Do the same process with the hips and heels against the wall to keep them in line.

6.   Parallel strapped position—try it sitting on the floor, bending and straightening legs (Figs. 11 and 12).

7.   Take straps off (Fig. 13).

2.   Effort — Shape: Rudolf Laban

Rudolf Laban was born in Austria in 1879 and died in London in 1958. He was an artist, scientist, architect, philosopher and movement educator. He observed the movement process in all aspects of life: from martial arts to factory work tasks, from dancers to emotionally disturbed people. The process of movement compelled his attention. He refined movement observation into an art that was used to make factories run more efficiently, record complicated ballets, and heal sick people.

Laban did not define "upright posture" as a static mechanism. To him it was a dynamic image—an ongoing, cohesive and three dimensional process that creates and recreates a series of relationships. He believed that even while "standing still" the whole body slightly sways in a figure eight path (the sign of infinity).

Observable phenomena can be looked at in terms of space, time, weight, and flow. Each of these has a yin and yang manifestation. (See Illus. 4.)

1. Space indications may be indirect (yin) or direct (yang).
2. Time may be sustained (yin) or quick (yang).
3. Weight or exertion may be light (yin) or strong (yang).
4. Flow may be free (yin) or bound (yang). Most people either struggle against or indulge in any motion. Movements with free flow cannot be easily interrupted or suddenly stopped; it takes time to gain control, whereas bound flow can be stopped at any instant.

The eight basic combinations of space, time, flow, and weight exertions by humans are (displayed by verbs to understand the movement)[2]:

Illus. 4

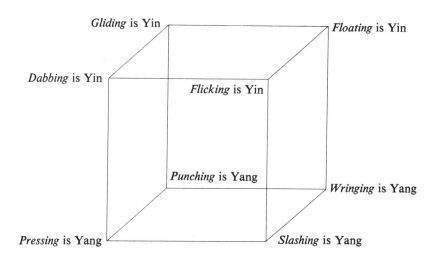

Process 2A:

Stand in the center of this box and reach to the eight corners doing the effort called for in each corner. Each basic effort has differentiations. For example, pressing includes crushing, squeezing, and cutting. We can see how useful this would be as a diagnostic tool: which efforts are strong, which are weak. The efforts on top may be described as more yin, and those on the bottom more yang.

These pieces of observable information may be put together in many ways to cure problems and understand many things. One can study the dances of a culture and understand their movement efforts, food and environment. Or watch the action of an emotionally disturbed person and discover what efforts are lacking. As you succeed in teaching the lacked effort, you will see the personality evolve. Another large field is applied to efficiency in work spaces (offices or factories).

One interesting story is of a cherry orchard. The buyers complained that the bottom layers of the crates of cherries were ripe but that the top layers were mixed with green and red. Carelessness was blamed on the workers. Movement observation showed regular and determined efforts at the beginning but later these efforts became erratic and undecided. It turned out that after a while the workers became temporarily color blind (red and green are complementary colors naturally confused by color blind people) and could not discern the ripe from the unripe. This made them run uncertainly from tree to tree. The cause of this disturbing irregularity was detected by observation of efforts characteristic of blind people. Color blind people often do not know that they are color blind. When the educators instructed the workers to relax their eyes periodically by looking at a neutral color, the problem ceased and the atmosphere of the work place was changed from one of restless discontent to peace.

A long-time student of Laban's work was Irmgard Bartenieff (born 1900, Berlin, died 1981, New York City). Her work deals with components of three major categories: 1) body, 2) space, and 3) effort, which are inexticably related in the movement process. The body has many components, expressions, givens, variables, and unknowns. Movement in space can be seen as taking place in the horizontal plane (side to side), vertical plane (up and down), or sagittal plane (front and back), taking place on a high, medium or low level. Any way of combining all these with three dimensional movements defines our kinesphere. Locomotion is moving the kinesphere: walking, running, stepping, rolling, somersaulting, crawling, sprinting, and all their variations.

> A movement makes sense only if it progresses organically, and this means that phrases which follow each other in a natural succession must be chosen.[3]
>
> —Laban

From that hypothesis Laban organized directional possibilities of movement and mobile shaping, and called them scales. They are related to geometric forms, which are like maps, and the scales are the route. He used octahedron, cube or *icosahedron* (visualized by superimposing the three planes on top of each other and connecting the peripheral points). Using these scales or movement sequences, the body would experience a wide range of efforts and shapes and spatial pulls.

Process 2B:

The reader may like to try a diagonal scale (one of the simpler ones).

Place yourself in the center of a cube, the limits of which are defined by your reaching:

1. high right forward (H.R.F.)
2. high right back (H.R.B.)
3. high left forward (H.L.F.)
4. high left back (H.L.B.)

and

1–4 all deep.

So the scale would be:

reach to

Illus. 5

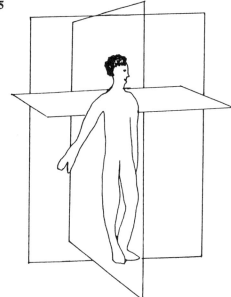

H.R.F. to	D.L.B.
D.L.B.	H.L.F.
H.L.F.	D.R.B.
D.R.B.	H.L.B.
H.L.B.	D.R.F.
D.R.F.	H.R.B.
H.R.B.	D.L.F.

The diagonal aim produces a slight twisting or spiral.

There are similarities between this exercise and the "cutting through delusions" exercise on page 121 of *The Book of Dō-In: Exercise for Physical and Spiritual Development* by Michio Kushi. The exercise consists of reaching from the upper right and cutting down with a sword (your hand) to the lower left. It is done on the diagonal in all directions and with a loud sound to dispel delusions in the form of mental-spiritual clouds of stagnation. I think that many modern exercises have grown out of these ancient spiritual practices that were intended to clear the spirit for a healthy life.

You may notice preferences, comforts, or difficulties in any diagonal. These may set up or limit your rhythm to move through the scale. Rhythm is an important factor in movement observation. Our vital functions—heartbeat and breath—have their own organized rhythm. On the other hand, exertion and recuperation activities, such as awake/asleep and work/rest are expressed more in spatial and effort patterns and use of body parts. All individuals and cultures have habitual phrasing of body movements, as we saw related to diet and life style.

Ms. Bartenieff worked for seven years in the polio ward at a New York hospital in the early 50s. The combination of training in physical therapy and Laban's work enabled her to get astonishing results. In her ward the immobilizing total body casts were replaced by special hot packs, which would help the stiffness in the back and neck. Along with Sister Kenny (an Australian nurse) she began to retrain individual muscles by awarensss and localization of their function.

One among many interesting stories: a four-year-old boy stricken with polio had been placed on a respirator for a few months, and as a result was left with a weak trunk, as well as weak arms and legs. Ms. Bartenieff began to expose him to all kinds of positions in space, such as tilting his torso or holding him upside-down. These activities evoked automatic reactions and reflexes, thus activating the spiralic musculature of the trunk to balance the body in all positions. Her focus was to restore his verticality and the ability to support his limbs from that verticality. This was in contrast to the traditional focus on muscular activity without spatial reference. After a few months he was able to sit in his crib. And ten months later he could walk with crutches and braces.

The emphasis was on total-body shaping and total-body mobility. Even if there is severe disability, the aim must be to reorder the fragmented patterns into a whole new form. The process proceeds by watching clues as one moves and not by imposing an end result (means whereby, not end-gaining). In my opinion, a macrobiotic diet combined with this movement would have helped the boy tremendously.

There are many more movement educators who have helped people begin to pay attention to their bodies. Among them are Moshe Feldenkrais, Bonnie Cohen, Milton Trager, Teachers of the *Reiki* Technique, Teachers of Tai Chi, Masahiro Oki, Bo In Lee, Yoga as taught by Iyengar and Swami Satchidananda, Ida Rolf, Ilana Rubenfeld, and many others who I do not know.

5. *Riding the Spirals of the Universe: Body Process Sequences*

"Certain exercises appear to stimulate thought. For this reason, perhaps, Aristotle and his disciples were in the habit of walking while discussing the fundamental problems of philosophy and science."[1]

—Alexis Carrel

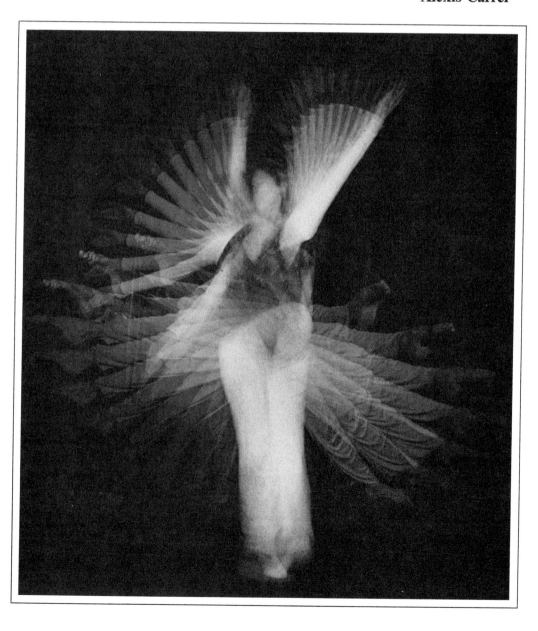

"Action and wisdom must be one."

—Masahiro Oki

I hesitate to use the word exercise as a chapter heading because that word has obligatory and negative connotations and implies mindless repetition. These sequences are designed to help anyone reach a deeper connection with themselves. They are not to develop any one set of muscles to be stronger than another.

My personal belief is that when the body is used, *treated*, and fed in accordance with its design, and a healthy, varied (not always sitting or driving, for example) active life is led, then not much extra attention is needed, for in that state, breathing tones, slightly stretches and stimulates (tonifies) all the muscles and this radiates out through the whole being. Since not many people live this way I will assume that in this stage of evolution these sequences will help many people to reclaim health and offset the damaging effects of our technologically advanced "life in the fast lane."

All of our learned movements are continually exposed to the possibility of becoming disordered to a major or minor degree at every stage in the learning process. In addition, any genetic, nutritional or environmental deficiency that any of us has suffered, either since infancy or due to accident or sickness, would leave its mark. Few, if any, civilized human beings have escaped these impacts.

Whether we arrive at it mechanically or reflexively, muscles and bones have certain directions or pulls and functions. The knee bends in one direction. If you try to bend it in the other direction (by pulling it back and hyperextending), you will eventually notice some trouble from the wrong pull.

How to use these sequences
If you come home exhausted from overwork, you may choose yin relaxing sequences to help you unwind and release excess tension. On the other hand, if you wake up feeling sluggish you may want to do purification sequences to wake up and stimulate yourself.

All must be done with an awareness of the primary controlling mechanism: the neck area must not be overly tense, so a coordinating action may take place throughout the organism. Between sequences all muscles return to neutral, a slightly stretched resting length, initiated by the spiralic torso muscles suspending the head.

For any lying down process, it is recommended to put a 2, 3, or 4 inch spacer under your head, so your head will not be back and down. All sequences are to be done without forgetting the breath, and with the face muscles relaxed. If you feel so inclined, a smile or the thought of a smile helps. The approach should include the spontaneity of a child at play coupled with the knowledge of conscious control.

These sequences grew out of many years of movement classes, study, meditation, and personal observations. I would like to give credit and thanks to Frances Cott, Bo In Lee, Masahiro Oki, Irmgard Bartenieff, David Gorman, F. M. Alexander, Raymond Dart, Tommy Thompson and Michio Kushi, for providing material for some of these sequences. As we saw in Chapter 1, "everything changes." My personal preference now (in 1986) is to teach the Alexander work and not the sequences.

With the diet and way of thinking that I am recommending, these sequences change so that individual sequences are not credited to specific teachers or methods. The

120

reader may try to 1) eat the diet, 2) train the mind, and 3) do the sequences. This may take away what you do not have (your delusions) and give you what you already have (your Buddha nature).

1. Breathing

When I told my four year old daughter that God is in all of us, she replied, "Anyway, how can he breathe inside there?"

"Breathing is not an activity but rather the result or response to an activity." That is why as we walk, jump, pray, or make love we breathe differently. We do not have to decide, "now I am running, so I will breathe faster"; it is a "built in" automatic response, a reflex. Breathing is the interchange between ourselves and the environment. Our harmonious adaptation to our environment is largely dependent on our breath.

The most important process or lesson to learn here is to allow the breath to respond. If we are not tightening or interfering and do not have actual physical blocks in the way, the air will come into us. When oxygen has been given and carbon dioxide taken out, the air will leave with no intervention by us. But if we are busy "posturing" or holding ourselves in a certain way, we may be preventing the breath from responding to the activity.

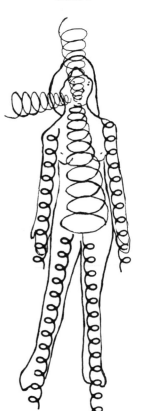

Illus. 1

As we ungrip all the muscles in the chest and around the ribs we create space, like a tiny vacuum, and the air rushes in to fill this. As you breathe out do not think of contracting, as is usually taught. As you exhale, be aware of the moment to moment freeing, creating the vacuum. As the old air leaves, the body immediately expands to open for new air. Again, this is "spiral thinking," where expansion and contraction meet.

As we watch water go down a drain, we see it traveling in a spiralic pattern. I assume the same phenomenon occurs with breath. If the mouth or nose is like the drain opening, the windpipe is the drain pipe and the air is like the water. Air will enter and travel in a spiral path (Illus. 1). This would only happen if we have emptied ourselves of doing or controlling. Illustration 2, a drawing made from a photograph taken inside the body, shows the spiralic pattern of smoke being sucked down into the lungs.[2]

As the neck is not tightening or closing the entrance, the breath enters and fills the lungs, and the ribs expand a bit in an upward direction if we are not actively pulling them (the ribs) down. Because the ribs are attached to the spine in the

Illus. 2

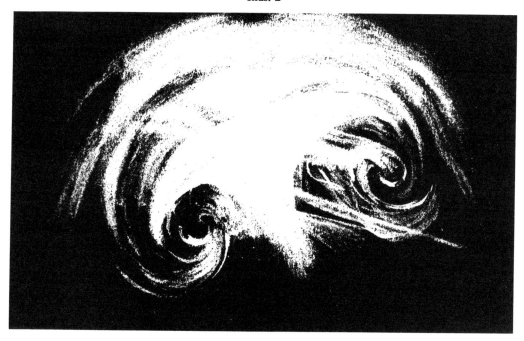

back by two synovial (freely moving) joints, as the ribs expand the spine lengthens a bit. Again, this occurs only if we are not busy holding it still in order to stand up straight. Then, as the whole torso is slightly expanded, the breath extends out the shoulders, down the arms to the hands and through the hip sockets, down the legs to the feet. As humans with free will we can stop it anywhere, consciously or unconsciously, and there will be no breath or air of life in that area. We do not want to set up a rigid breathing pattern or habit but we must allow the present moment and conditions to adjust each breath.

Because our systems are interdependent, our way of breathing affects not only the respiratory but also the circulatory, excretory, and nervous systems. Active, alive breathing accelerates and stimulates these systems, as well-functioning systems allow active full breath. The same may be said about slow, inactive breath, leading to slow organ function and vice versa. The important understanding of breath cannot be overstated, because breath affects all organs and functions, as well as emotional states, thoughts and spiritual conditions.

There are many techniques for breath control to direct the breath to one place or another. These are used to restore the body to a state of balance or to travel to some particular state or consciousness. As a sales person, if you adopt the same breathing and movement patterns as your client, you can sell them anything. Since breath is an automatic muscular response, too many conscious attempts to control it may prove dangerous to your health. It is important to remember while practicing these techniques not to forsake the whole for a part.

122

Process 1A: Heaven and Earth

We may use the breath to accelerate already existing directions of movement.

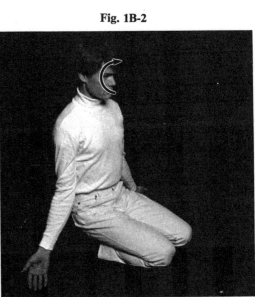

Fig. 1A

1. Breathe in upward (earth's force) (Fig. 1A). This stimulates the nervous system and upward blood flow and provides an overall lifted feeling.

2. Breathe out (heaven's force) to stimulate the digestive system, downward blood flow, and motion toward the earth. Steps 1 and 2 activate heaven's energy and earth's energy.

3. There are many varieties of this type of breathing. Another example: breathe into the sixth chakra or third eye, breathe out to the second chakra or *hara* (two fingers below navel).

Process 1B: Yin and Yang

You can breathe continuously, accenting one direction or the other, creating yin or yang conditions.

1. Yang:

Breathe into the hara, hold several seconds, make the exhalation 2 to 3 times longer (Fig. 1B-1). Hands on lap. Grounded feelings, stability. Get warmer. Faster breath—quicker metabolism. Narrow perception to parts. Used for martial arts to create strength for the physical center of the body.

2. Yin:

Fig. 1B-1

Fig. 1B-2

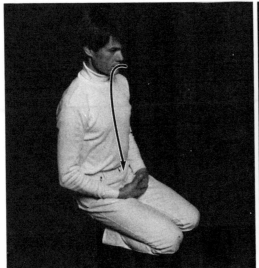

Breathe up to forehead slowly and continuously, then release out through mouth (Fig. 1B-2). Open hands at sides. Consciousness floats. Get cooler. Slower breath —metabolism slows. Wider perception of the whole. Used in many religious practices to release the body attachment and to free into the spiritual world.

Fig. 1C

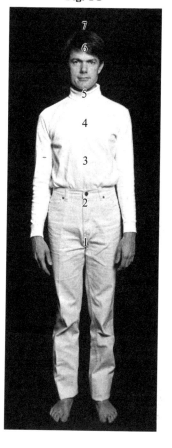

Process 1C: Chakra Characteristics

1. We can send breath to each of the chakras to stimulate the area and their characteristics (Fig. 1C).
   7—Entrance of heaven's force—universal understanding
   6—Insight, wisdom
   5—Oneness with atmosphere
   4—Emotional harmony
   3—Intellect and coordination
   2—Physical stability
   1—Entrance of earth's force—adaptability

Process 1D: Acupuncture Pathways

We can send breath through acupuncture pathways (meridians) to clear blocks that may occur, or to stimulate a certain organ. One example would be the Conception Vessel and the Governing Vessel.

1. Breathe in—air goes up the spine, over the top head, and into the mouth; Breathe out—down through the torso; Breathe in—up the front of the body and into

Fig. 1D

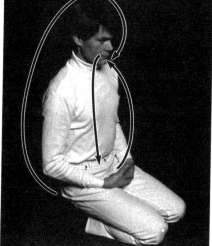

Illus. 3

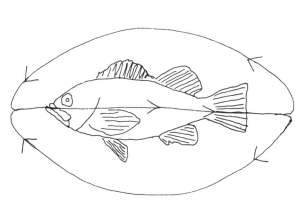

the mouth; Breathe out—down through the torso. Continue. (Illus. 3 and Fig. 1D)

Followers of certain Buddhist sects in Japan believe that because of its unifying qualities this style practiced one half hour a day will cure all problems. Note that the torso has up and down motion but the head only has forward and upward direction. These people intuitively understood what Alexander later put into words. "He became known as the 'breathing man' and people wanted to know how he did it," Walter Carrington said of F. M. Alexander.[3]

Process 1E: Breathing Awareness

1. Breathe into your upper chest. Hold for two counts and let out quickly all the way down to the very bottom of your torso. Notice where the breath does not go.

2. Breathe in all directions. Take a partner. Put a hand anywhere on your partner's body and say, "Breathe into my hand." Notice to what part of the body the breath does not flow readily.

3. On the floor on your back breathe so your ribs open sideways and not forward and back. Put your hands on the sides of ribs, fingers down. On inhale lift sides of ribs up. Breathe out, release.

4. Breathing is the most complete exercise done all the time, affecting all parts. Breathing excites and moves energy. Energy breaks blocks of tension (tightened muscles). Blocking causes heaviness. Breathing creates lightness. Breathe out more than you breathe in to keep the system slightly alkaline. The out breath can be thought of as the letting go of past ideas, thoughts or holdings that we no longer need. The in breath is the new, fresh energy for beginning.

5. To see the power of the breath, if your mood is uncomfortable check which nostril you are breathing out of. To change the mood, close that one and breathe through the other for a minute or so.

2. Awareness of Total Body

Process 2A: Directions

Anyone at any time can benefit from taking a few moments to listen to his or her body. The messages or signals are all there. We just have to listen to them.

To Begin: Lie down on the floor with a 2, 3, or 4 inch book supporting your head. Your knees should be bent so that your feet are flat on the floor near your buttocks and the hands are on your abdomen, with elbows by your sides (Fig. 2A).

1. Begin to observe, *without doing anything*, aches, sensations, holdings or tension. Observe yourself in relationship to your environment (eyes open).

2. Then again without doing anything think of allowing your neck to be free.

3. As the neck is free from holding, the head moves slightly forward and up.

4. As this happens, let the spine ever so lightly lengthen and widen.

Fig. 2A

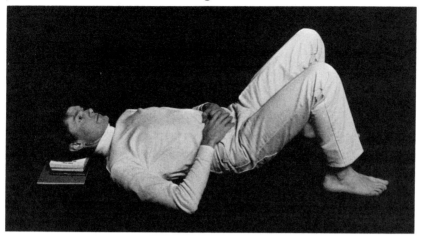

5.   Then allow the upper arms to widen, the elbows to free down away from the body, and the forearms to free away from the wrists. Hands are free and empty.

6.   The ribs are left alone to expand for breathing. The abdomen, jaw and anus are not held.

7.   The hip sockets are let go. The knees free upward toward the ceiling and the heels free into the floor. The feet not gripping.

8.   The whole body is supported by the floor (or earth's energy and the spatial suspension).

9.   Again check where the tensions are in relationship to this and where the breath does not go. My muscles have excess tension because I am holding them, consciously or unconsciously. To continue, *I* can stop the holding (inhibition). I do so not by releasing specific muscles but by staying with the primary control steps 2–4. This sequence is based on the "directions or orders" established by F. M. Alexander. A qualified Alexander teacher is able to give this experience in movement (an experience I highly recommend). Practicing this regularly one may cultivate an awareness that enhances all aspects of life.

Process 2B: On Stomach

1.   Another position to try would be the prone, lying on the stomach with forehead on the floor and a pillow under the breast bone (if needed). Arms by your sides, palms up (Fig. 2B-1). This allow the nerves in your head and your body balancing senses to relax.

Fig. 2B-1

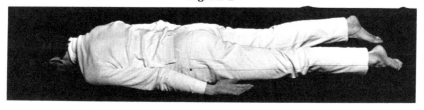

126

Fig. 2B-2

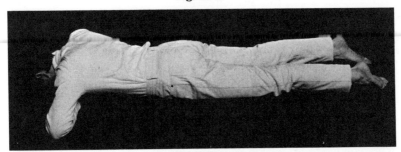

Fig. 2B-3

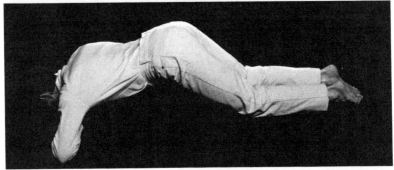

Fig. 2B-4

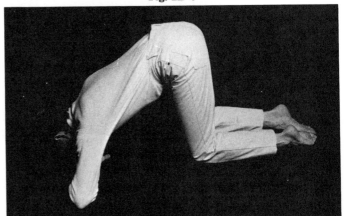

Fig. 2B-5

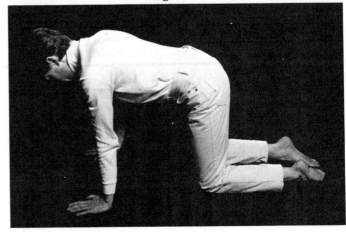

2. After you can lie here and breathe comfortably begin to slowly move first your head, then your torso and limbs. This is the first and safest of all ancestral positions for a terrestrial vertebrate.

3. Then you can begin to roll over by pressing the back of one hand or foot into the floor. Note the tensions and adjustments in your head and body as you do this. Play with the observations and roll over when you are ready.

4. You may then try lying on your stomach with your hands under your breast bone (Fig. 2B-2). Try to lift the chest from the forehead and elbows and continue breathing regularly (Fig. 2B-3).

5. Once this is mastered try drawing the knees up to their body supporting position as you are breathing regularly (Fig. 2B-4). From here we can explore many ways to stand, keeping in mind the freedom of your head-neck-body relationship, and the awareness of your environment.

6. One position along the way would be crawling. Begin on the hands and knees (Fig. 2B-5). Allow the head to move forward into space and then when necessary the limbs (arms and legs) will move to support the torso. (In motion, Fig. 2B-6.)

Fig. 2B-6

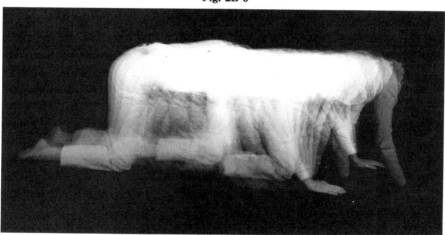

Process 2C: Chakra Movement

Each chakra may be used to produce and develop a different quality.

7) Crown—develops universal understanding (brain)

Fig. 2C

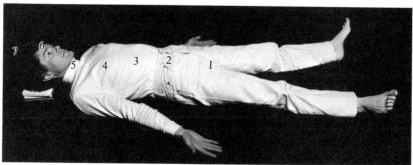

128

6) Forehead—develops wisdom and spiritual understanding (nervous system)
5) Throat—develops expression (mouth and lungs)
4) Heart—develops emotional perception and harmony (circulatory system)
3) Solar Plexus—develops coordination and reasoning (central digestive organs)
2) Sacral—develops life power and stability (intestines)
1) Base—develops adaptability and reproduction (excretory and reproductive)
1. Start lying down or standing (Fig. 2C).
2. No tension in the neck.
3. Take breath and energy first to the base chakra.
4. Continue 3. Allow natural movement to occur and then carry you through space.
5. Stop and center yourself, no tension in the neck, and do the next chakra. Continue through the crown.

Process 2D: Expand-contract

Start curled in a ball as small as you can be (Fig. 2D-1). Open from the inside to out (yang to yin) so that the central torso opens first and arms and legs extend last, as you spiral up to standing. Fill as much space as you can beyond hands into the sky, and below feet into the earth (Fig. 2D-2). This is not an image but a reality. Your vibration does extend like this. You are: from the single cell, to organs, to systems, the physical whole you, your immediate surroundings, your large environment, your country, the world, the galaxy, the universe, the infinite.

Fig. 2D-1

Fig. 2D-2

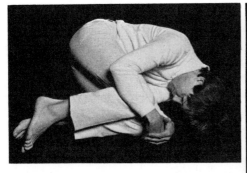
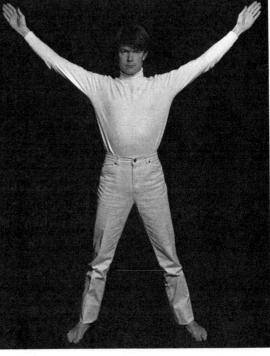

Then back, through all the stages to the ball on the floor. The body folds in horizontally and vertically all at once. Sequentially gather the parts of the body into a central point. First the closest to the center torso, and then the periphery comes in last. Be sure that arms and legs move and rotate sequentially and not all in one piece.

3. Walking

Because the physical body as a whole is a suspension system, all muscles are extended with equal tensional balance supporting each other. We must continue to coordinate this unity as we move into space (Fig. 3).

Let us start with the idea that the head leads and the body follows. The senses in the head seek, and the body is ordered accordingly. In a walk, because we want to move forward we must release the neck muscles to allow the head to move forward. Because of that release there is a slight rise in the whole head.

As the head is allowed to move slightly forward and up this extends a slight stretch along the spine. As there is a bit more space between the vertebrae to give more length, the ribs (attached to the vertebrae) also get more space for more width.

As this slight lift takes place the leg is free to move in the hip socket starting with a release of the knee forward. The three major moveable joints in the legs release for movement—knee, hip and ankle.

The spiral muscles in the torso that we have discussed form a support system for moving. As we walk one spiral expands while another contracts.

Fig. 3

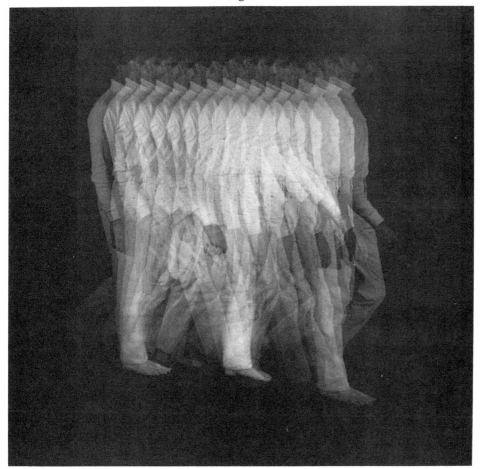

Process 3A: Spirals Walking

Fig. 3A

1. To get a sense of this, have a friend take two pieces of rope about 3 to 4 feet long. Put one end on the left hip crest. Go diagonally up to the right bottom of the rib cage, around the back and up to the left side of the skull (Fig. 3A). Do the other side. Sense (a) the whole of the foot over the whole of the ground and (b) the ground supporting you. Then release the head up into freedom as the body follows, and release the knee to move. Experiment with all the double helix spiral patterns (in Chapter 1).

Many people start to walk by leaning down somewhere: in the foot, hip, or lower back. They are consistently lifting themselves up from this falling down. They have to react to the fall plus move themselves forward in space. This is usually accompanied by some set in the torso, preventing an overall "up" integrity of unity. We would like the neck-free reflex, followed by the intention to move, guide the walk. This works provided we are not posturing the torso muscles (to look like Marlon Brando, or Marilyn Monroe).

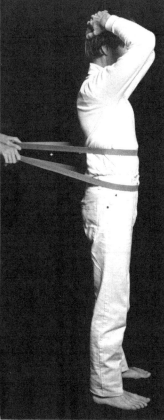

Fig. 3B-1   Fig. 3B-2

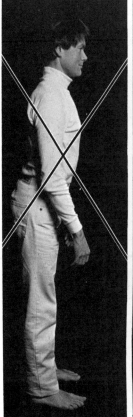

Process 3B: Retrain Walk

1.   Many people walk by first contracting their lower back, or pushing their pelvic crests or chest forward (Fig. 3B-1).

To help retrain this habit put a rope around A's lower ribs and top hip crest and stand behind him. As A walks, keeping in mind the head neck relationship, B does not allow the front ribs or front hip crests to lead (Fig. 3B-2).

A few things to watch out for:

a.   Toes and foot spread over whole floor, they do not grip. The foot has many movable parts to adapt to the surface.

b. Heel leads down to lengthen calf.
c. Ankle bones do not roll in.
d. Knees never "lock" back.
e. Pelvis does not drop back to move.
f. Bottom of rib cage does not stick out to lead.
g. Head does not drop back.
h. Three major joints (ankle, knee, and hip) are not held stiff.
(In motion, walk arms up Fig. 3B-3.)

Fig. 3B-3

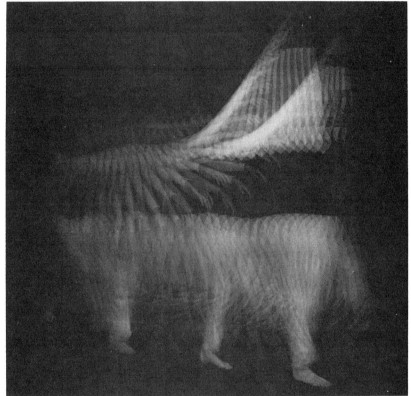

4. Diagonals

Many of these diagonal sequences begin on the floor in an X position. This means that there is a straight diagonal line from the left hand to the right foot and from the right hand to left foot. If possible have a friend check your overview to make sure that the pulls are even.

In these sequences we are stimulating the oblique or diagonal muscles. This set supports our spiralic structure and provides an internal supporting latticework from which we move. Figures 4-1 and 4-2 show left and right of one set of diagonals.

Figure 4-3 shows another set of diagonals in the length of the torso.

Fig. 4-1 Fig. 4-2 Fig. 4-3

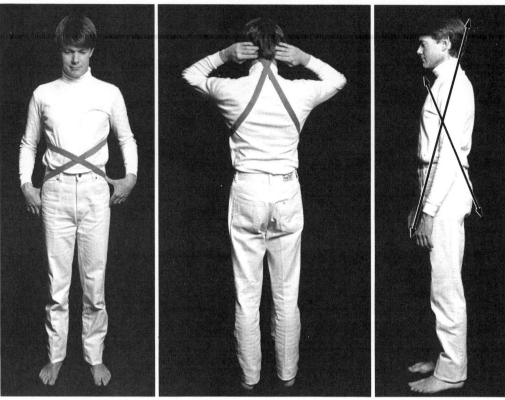

a. One from the coccyx to the sternum
b. One from the pubic bone to the mastoid process

I recommend no standard situps because they strengthen the vertical abdominals which are not best suited for building support in that area (explained in Chapter 4, Section 4). To get an idea of these spirals, lie on the floor on your back with knees bent. Keeping your lower back on the floor, twist your shoulders one way and knees another. Try the other side. I do not speak of stretching any muscles because that has been found to tear muscle fibers. I advise "yield," not "stretch."

Process 4A: Knee to Elbow Spiral-up

1. Lie on the floor, body in X hand to foot (Fig. 4A-1). Do not lock joints.
2. Breathe in and extend left arm and right foot.
3. Breathe out and simultaneously circle left elbow down and right knee up (Figs. 4A-2–4).
4. They meet (Fig. 4A-5). Middle body sinks to the floor. Working but not knotted in stomach. Cycle feeling.
5. Breathe in, and on out breath, shoot knee and elbow back to floor (Fig. 4A-1).
6. Other side. (In motion, Fig. 4A-6).

Fig. 4A-1

Fig. 4A-2

Fig. 4A-3

Fig. 4A-4

Fig. 4A-5

Fig. 4A-6

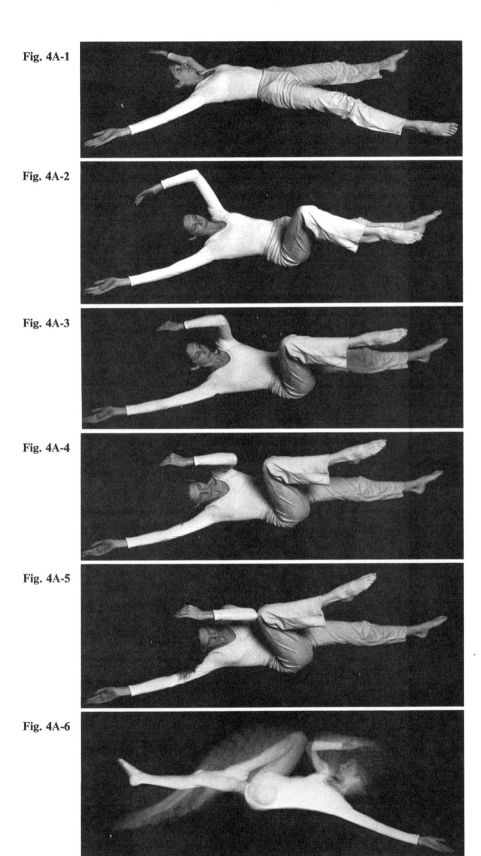

Process 4B: Diagonal Spiral Up from Fetal

1. Lie in fetal position on left side (Fig. 4B-1).
2. Begin to open body, extend right leg back, and circle right arm overhead (Fig. 4B-2).
3. Pass through X on floor (Fig. 4B-3).
4. Bring left hand toward right hand (Fig. 4B-4).
5. End fetal on right side (Fig. 4B-5). Repeat to other side. *Variation:* repeat 4B-1–4.
6. Continue reaching left hand along the floor until the left hand reaches right foot (Fig. 4B-6).
7. Continue the right hand to the left foot (Fig. 4B-7).
8. Continue reaching, making a large circle on the floor with the arm and spiral back down (Figs. 4B-8 and 9).
9. Pass through X (Fig. 4B-10).

10. End fetal (Figs. 4B-11 and 12). Other side. (In motion, Figure 4B-13.)

Move on the out breath. Use the oblique muscles, not the verticals. This may be incorporated into your daily life. As you get up from a lying down on your back position, it is less strain to turn on your side and spiral up.

Fig. 4B-1

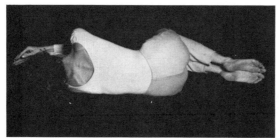

Fig. 4B-2

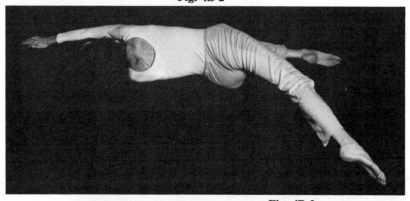

Fig. 4B-3

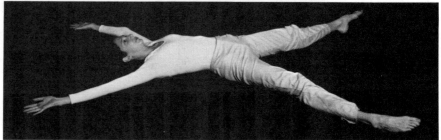

Fig. 4-B4

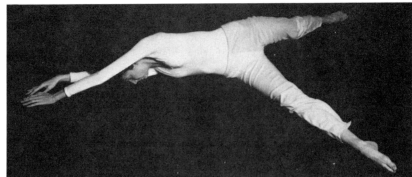

Fig. 4B-5

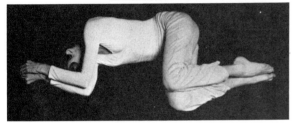

Fig. 4B-6

Fig. 4B-7

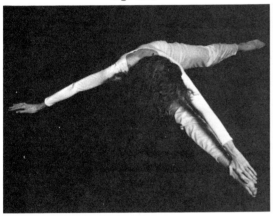
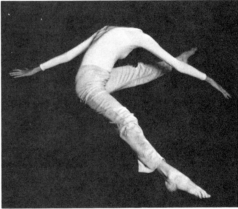

Fig. 4B-8

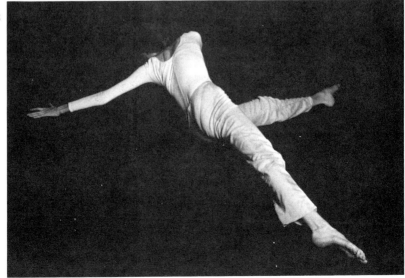

136

Fig. 4B-9

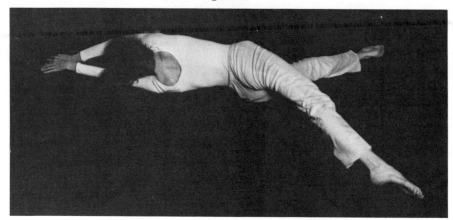

Fig. 4B-10

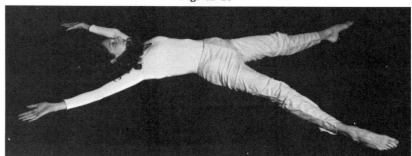

Fig. 4B-11

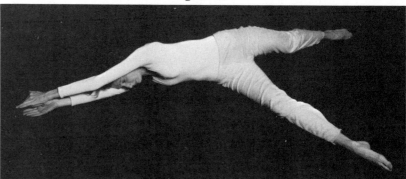

Fig. 4B-12

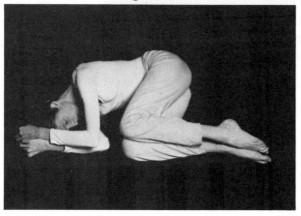

Fig. 4B-13

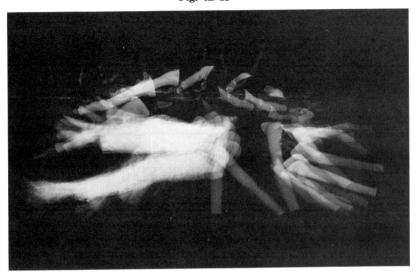

Process 4C: Diagonal Spiral Up from X

1. Begin in X on the floor (Fig. 4C-1).
2. Extend and spiral out right hand (Fig. 4C-2).

Fig. 4C-1

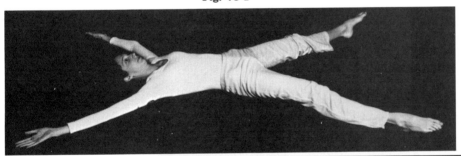

Fig. 4C-2

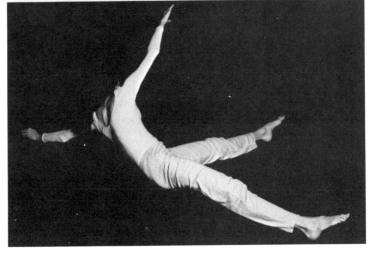

138

Fig. 4C-3

Fig. 4C-4

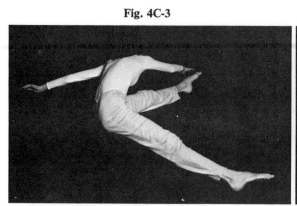
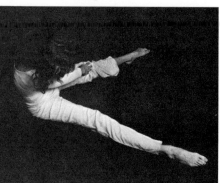

Fig. 4C-5

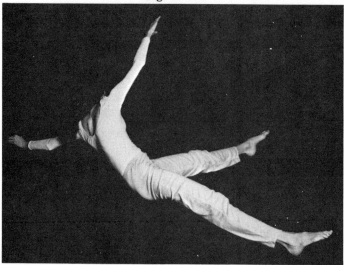

Fig. 4C-6

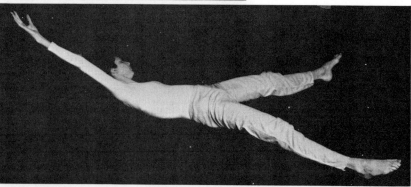

Fig. 4C-7

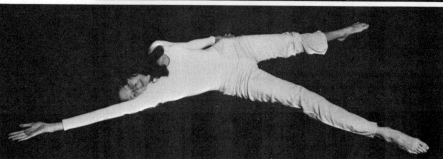

3. Right hand reaches up and over to left foot. Body has slight spiral to left side. Hand makes a big curve over to foot (Fig. 4C-3). Be sure to stay on the diagonal line.

4. Return on the diagonal so that you end off of your X center (Figs. 4C-4–7).

Process 4D: Leg Turnover

1. Lie on stomach in X (Fig. 4D-1).

2. Reach out through left toes. Raise the left leg toward right foot and continue reaching left foot until it turns you over on your back (Figs. 4D-2–5).

3. Then left foot reaches toward right foot to get you back to starting X (Figs. 4D-6–10). Other side.

Fig. 4D-1

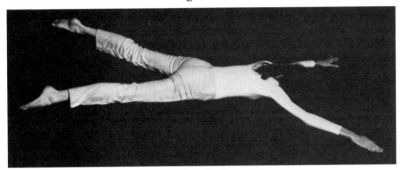

Fig. 4D-2

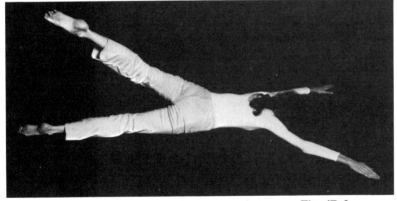

Fig. 4D-3

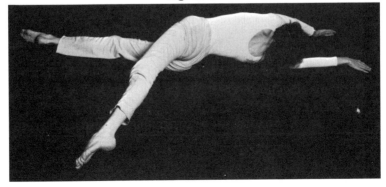

140

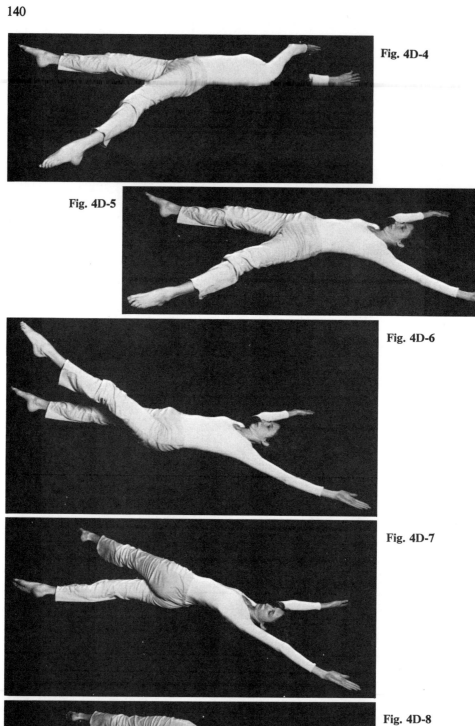

Fig. 4D-4

Fig. 4D-5

Fig. 4D-6

Fig. 4D-7

Fig. 4D-8

Don't arch lower back. Try the same process beginning lying on your back with your foot leading. Try it taking the leg as high as possible or as close to the ground as possible.

Fig. 4D-9

Fig. 4D-10

Fig. 4E-1

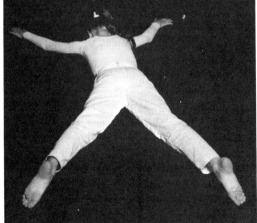

Process 4E: Arm Turnover
(Same as leg turnover, but with arm)

1. Lie on stomach in X shape (Fig. 4E-1).
2. Bring left hand slightly off the ground and move it toward right (Fig. 4E-2).
3. Keep reaching arm until you turn over (Figs. 4E-3 and 4). Arm leads over, not shoulder. Keep a straight line, toe to hand, sink lower back to floor. Don't arch lower back. Don't let hip come readily.

Fig. 4E-2

Fig. 4E-3

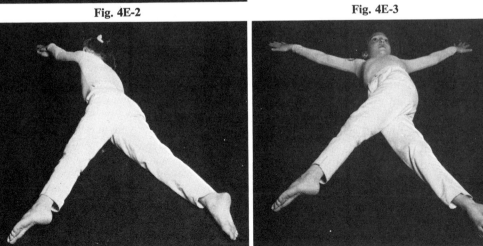

142

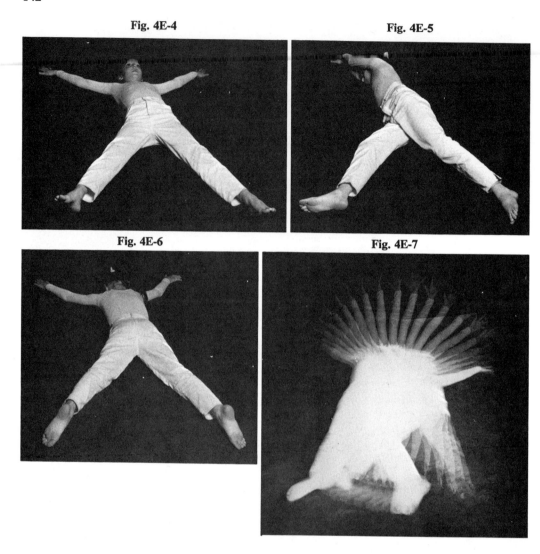

Fig. 4E-4   Fig. 4E-5

Fig. 4E-6   Fig. 4E-7

4.   Left hand and arm lead over and land on your stomach in X (Figs. 4E-5 and 6). Other side. (In motion, Figure 4E-7.) Try it starting on your back.

Process 4F: Back Turnover

1.   Lie in X on the floor on your back (Fig. 4F-1).
2.   On out breath bring right knee to left shoulder until you end up on your

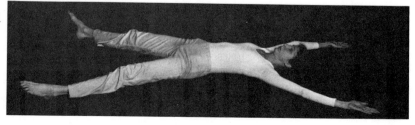

Fig. 4F-1

stomach (Figs. 4F-2–8). Let leg drop; push through right heel to straighten. Press left heel to floor.

3. Leg follows same path to return. Right knee toward left shoulder (Figs. 4F-9–11). Allow middle back to hit first by curving the torso.

4. Return to X (Fig. 4F-12). Other side.

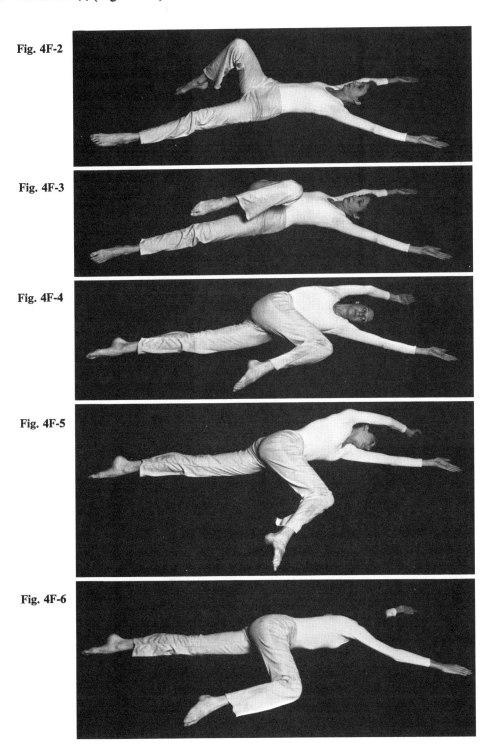

Fig. 4F-2

Fig. 4F-3

Fig. 4F-4

Fig. 4F-5

Fig. 4F-6

144

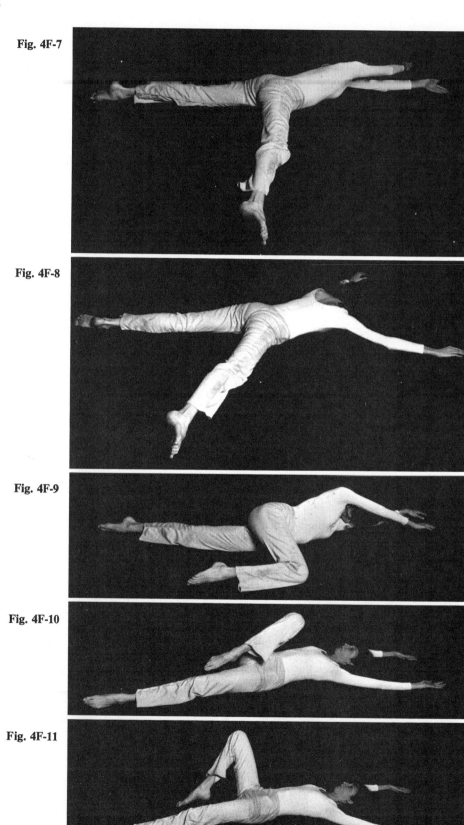

Fig. 4F-7

Fig. 4F-8

Fig. 4F-9

Fig. 4F-10

Fig. 4F-11

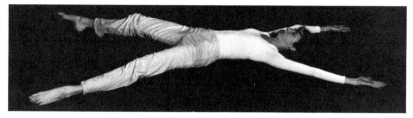

Fig. 4F-12

Process 4G: Arm Spiral Up

1.   Lie on the floor, arms horizontal, knees bent, and breathe (Fig. 4G-1).
2.   Drop knees to right side. Move left arm up to make diagonal to left knee (Fig. 4G-2).

Fig. 4G-1

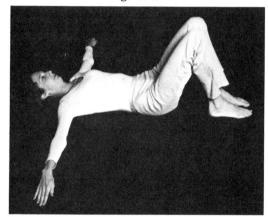

Fig. 4G-2

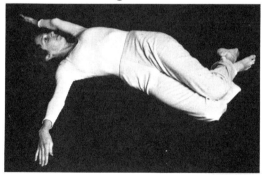

3.   Left arm begins to circle *overhead*. Rotate arm in a circle around body reaching out through fingertips and keeping hand on the floor as long as possible (Figs. 4G-3–6). Circle arm three times.

4.   Then build speed in left arm movement and momentum takes you up (Figs. 4G-7–9).

5.   Continue right arm to make a circle around you and your body spirals back down to the left side (Figs. 4G-10–13).

6.   Right arm circles overhead to return (Figs. 4G-14–16).

Keep that hand really reaching and when you go down you won't hit the floor hard. The arm is supported by the floor. It starts going over your head. Increase spatial tension. Increase diameter—don't skip places in the circle. Don't make yourself come up. Your body decides when for you if spatial tension is right.

Fig. 4G-3

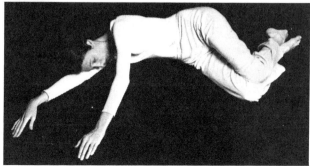

146

Fig. 4G-4

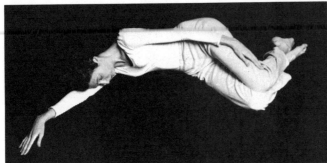

Fig. 4G-5

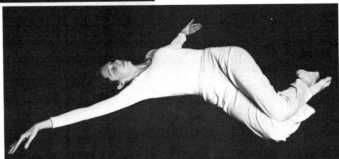

Fig. 4G-6

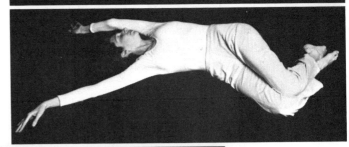

Fig. 4G-7

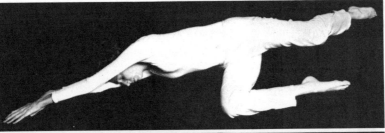

Fig. 4G-8

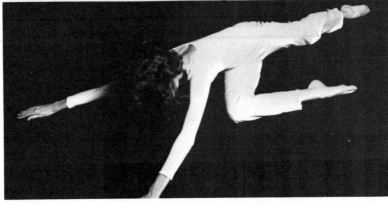

147

Fig. 4G-9

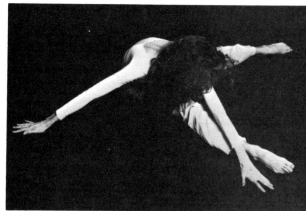

Fig. 4G-10

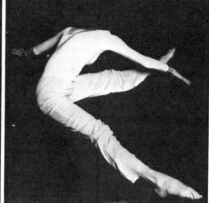

Fig. 4G-11

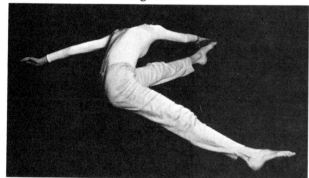

Fig. 4G-12

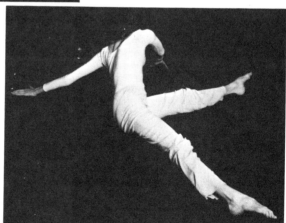

Fig. 4G-13

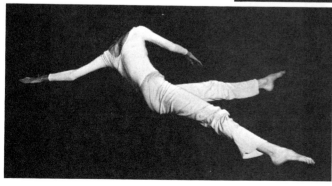

Fig. 4G-14

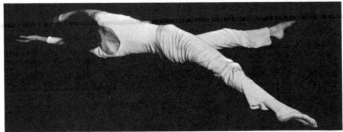

Fig. 4G-15

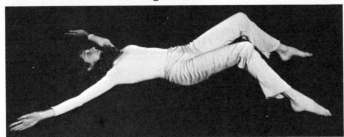

Fig. 4G-16

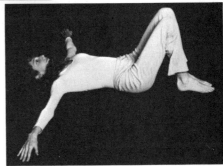

Process 4H: Spiral Up to Standing

Begin in X on floor (Fig. 4H-1).

1.   Left leg comes over to cross right leg (as if over a barrel) and place foot on the floor (Fig. 4H-2). Return to X (Fig. 4H-1).

Fig. 4H-1

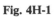
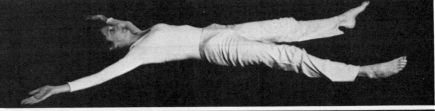

Fig. 4H-2

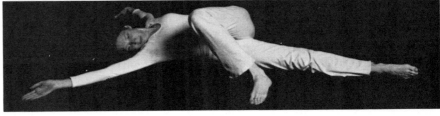

2. Left hand and foot reach over body and place on floor (Fig. 4H-3). Return to X (Fig. 4H-1).

3. Repeat 2 and lift head as hands and foot reach for the floor (Fig. 4H-4). Return to X (Fig. 4H-1).

4. Repeat 3 and lift pelvis as hand and foot reach for the floor (Fig. 4H-5). Return to X (Fig. 4H-1).

5. Repeat steps 1 to 4 and continue to move your body in the direction of spiral until you stand (Figs. 4H-6–9).

6. Then spiral body back down in the direction from which you came and return to X.

7. Repeat steps 1 to 5. Continue to stand and keep going in that same direction and spiral down back to X (Figs. 4H-10–15). Other side. (In motion, Figure 4H-16.)

Ride your spiral waves with a smile.

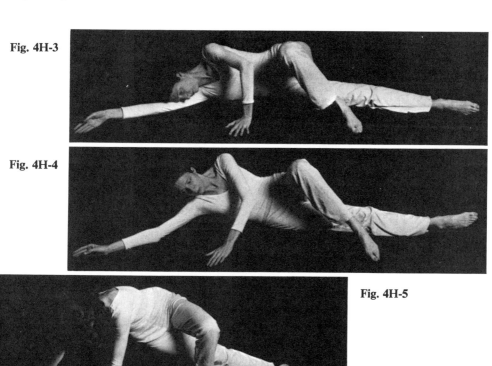

Fig. 4H-3

Fig. 4H-4

Fig. 4H-5

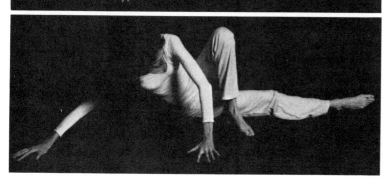

Fig. 4H-6

150

Fig. 4H-7

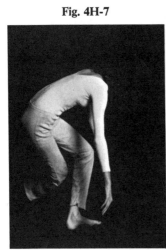

Fig. 4H-8

Fig. 4H-9

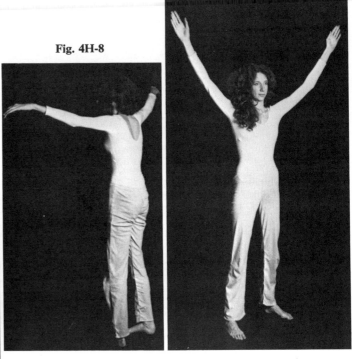

Fig. 4H-10

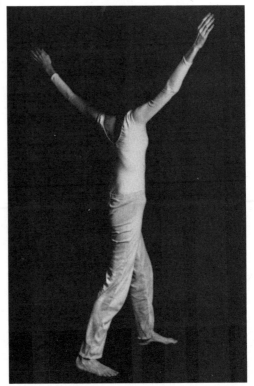

151

Fig. 4H-11

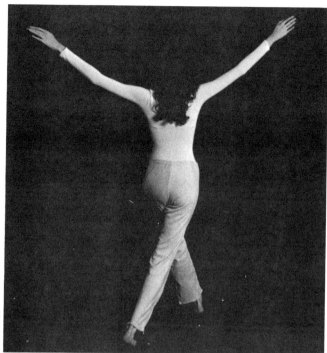

Fig. 4H-12

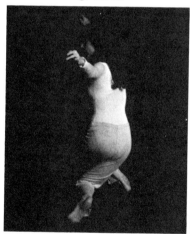

Fig. 4H-13

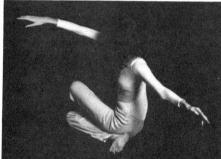

Fig. 4H-14

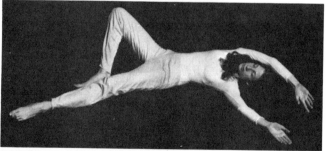

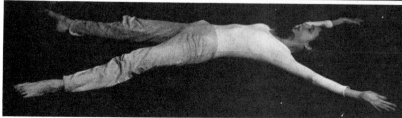

Fig. 4H-15

Fig. 4H-16

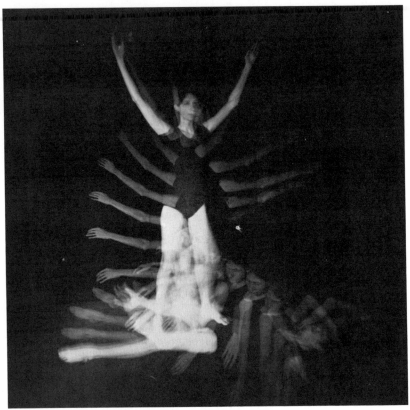

5. Spatial Tension

Spatial tension is a *slight* lengthening between two parts. One part stretches away while the other part gently resists. A pull in two directions, freeing toward each other and away at the same time.

Process 5A: Spatial Tension Sitting

1. Sit on the floor. Buttocks on heels and arms over head.
2. Feel axis of spatial tension from coccyx to top head and lean it: a) forward (Fig. 5A-1), b) side (Fig. 5A-2), c) back, d) side (Fig. 5A-3), and e) anywhere off center. But do not bend your body, keep the axis straight and head forward and up.

Process 5B: Spatial Tension Moving

1. Start standing. Arms overhead with spatial tension between feet and hands.

Fig. 5A-1   Fig. 5A-2   Fig. 5A-3

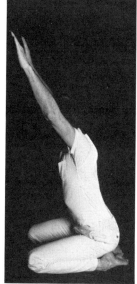 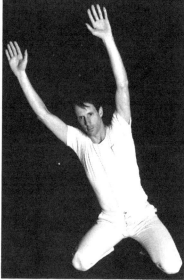 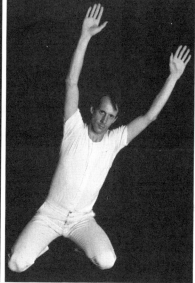

Fig. 5B

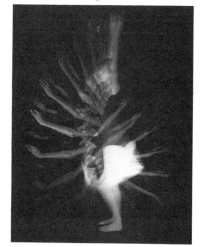

2.   On the out breath reach arms forward until body bends over and bend knees. A "let go" feeling.

3.   Then straighten knees as arms reach behind body. Return to step 2, then 1. (In motion, Fig. 5B.) After you can build momentum, jump on 1 and 3 and 1 and 3, and so on.

Process 5C: Diagonal Spatial Tension

1.   Start standing, reaching left and right hands to right side diagonal and left foot to left diagonal with spatial tension between hands and left foot.

Fig. 5C-1   Fig. 5C-2

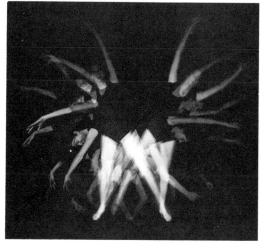 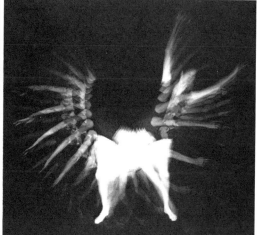

2. Reach right and left arm to right side and circle to center as you drop body (especially head) in center of body and bend knees (let go feeling).

3. Continue reaching arms to left side and let them lead you to standing, reaching to left side diagonal as right foot points to right side diagonal (Fig. 5C-1).

Repeat to other side. In motion, Figure 5C-2.

Process 5D: Spatial Tension Traveling

When this is comfortable and the momentum is smooth you may try it traveling across the floor as the arms swing.

1. Reach arms to the right side.
2. Drop arms center as you step to left.
3. Arms reach up and circle overhead as momentum lifts you off the ground.
4. Arms continue to swing over to left side. In motion, Figure 5D.

The dance continues, the dancer disappears.

Fig. 5D

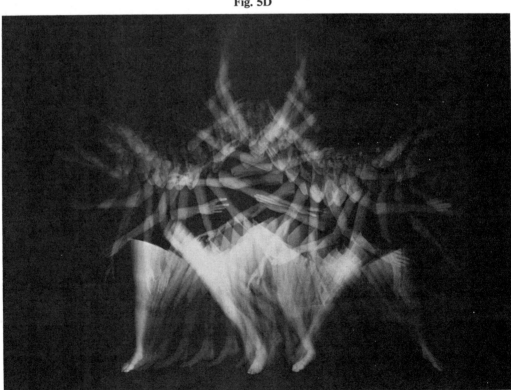

6. Arms

Process 6A: General Arm Tension

1. Take a small rubber ball 3 inches diameter, place it between the shoulder blades and lie down on your back and relax. This helps the chest to open so that the arms can free out. You may vary size, and hardness and placement of ball (Fig. 6A).

Fig. 6A

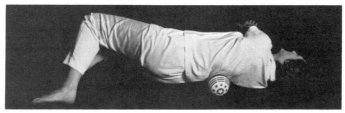

Process 6B: Elbow Stretch

Place elbow on towel on a ledge and pull hand out (Fig. 6B).

Fig. 6B

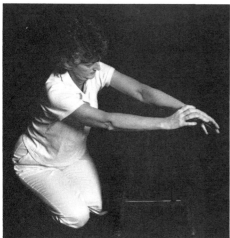

Fig. 6C

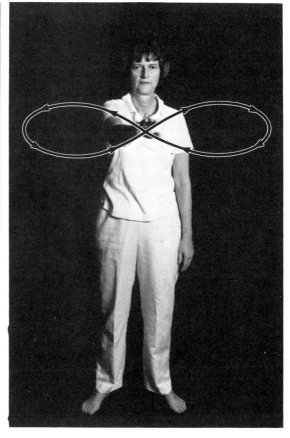

Process 6C: Figure eight

Stand and make a figure eight with one hand in front of you (Fig. 6C). Make both sides even. Use the rotation in the joints in the arms. The back of hand leads down on both sides. Do it on the horizontal. Then do it on the vertical—keep arm rotation—up and down. Let arm moving in figure eight take you in any direction. Move it across the floor. Turn limbs in and out.

Fig. 6D-1

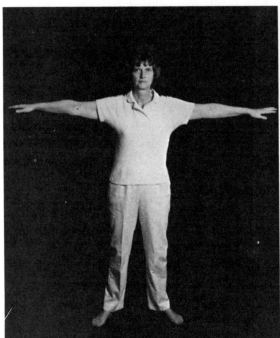

Fig. 6D-2

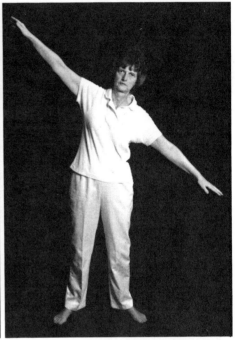

Fig. 6D-3

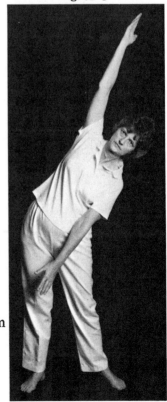

Process 6D: Synchronize Two Arms

1.   Standing, start arms out to the sides (Fig. 6D-1).
2.   Reach one arm over the top of your head while the other makes an opposite pull by your thighs (Fig. 6D-2).
3.   Keep the diagonal pull. Be sure to have equal pull in both hands (Fig. 6D-3). Allow body to tilt slightly in the direction of pull. Keep collar bone area open, and neck free.

Process 6E: Swing Arms

1.   Start arms to left side (Fig. 6E-1).
2.   Swing to right side (Fig. 6E-2).
3.   Return (Fig. 6E-3).
4.   Then swing arms to the right so that the momentum carries you and you take two steps to turn around (Fig. 6E-4). End arms to right side. Allow the swing of the arms to carry the movement. Other side. In motion, Figure 6E-5.

157

Fig. 6E-1

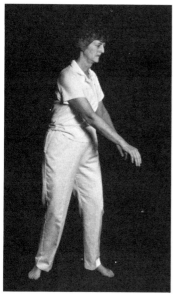

Fig. 6E-2

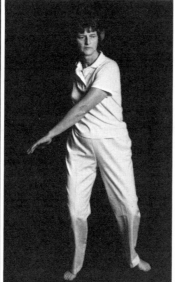

Fig. 6E-3

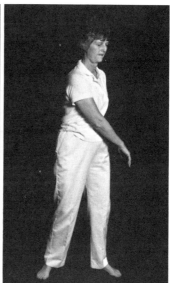

Fig. 6E-4

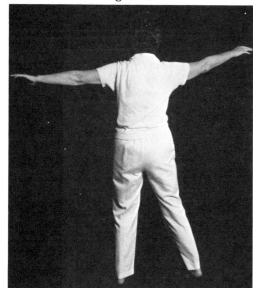

Fig. 6E-5

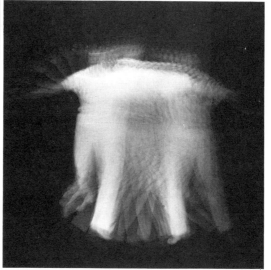

Process 6F: Hand Meridians

Figure 6F-1.

Fig. 6F

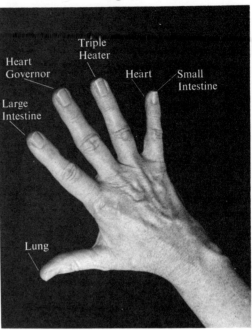

Fig. 6F

7. To Unfold Leg

Fig. 7A-1   Fig. 7A-2

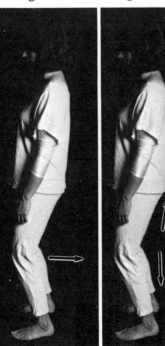

Instead of thinking about "straightening the leg" let us think of "unfolding the leg." "To straighten a leg" has connotations to mean pull the calf back and tense the thigh.

Process 7A: How to Unfold Leg

If a leg is bent there are two ways to make it straight.

1. Push the calf back until it is straight, often creating hyperextension or an "s" curve in the leg (Fig. 7A-1).

2. Stabilize the foot over the floor and lift the hips up from the top. Ideally this is set up by the freedom of the head-neck-back relationship (Fig. 7A-2).

If you practice step 1, you set up wrong forces or zigzags of muscle pulls, whereas step 2

159

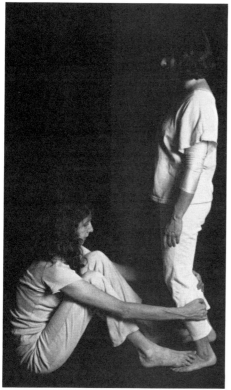

Fig. 7B

harmonizes the actions of the body to the legs. You don't want to "pull" the pelvis up from top with strong muscular contractions. You don't want to push it up from below. You want to release any pulling or holding that might be preventing the upward spiralic motion. There are no front and back mechanical pulls to unfold a leg.

Process 7B: Stabilize Foot and Move Buttocks

1.   A stands with bent knees, hips over heels. (Fig. 7B). B holds calves of A.
2.   A straightens legs from the top length and has no back pressure in calves. Gluteus comes back and up. For more stretch do it against the wall. Stand bent over with your back on the wall, knees bent and feet close to wall. Lift buttocks to straighten. Do not pull calves back.

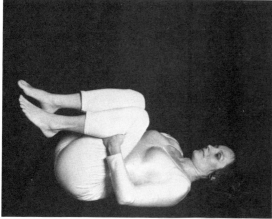

Fig. 7C-1

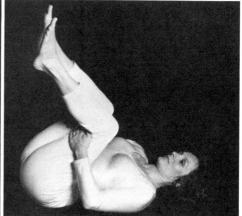

Fig. 7C-2

Process 7C: Stabilize Buttocks and Move Foot

Lie on the floor on your back (Fig. 7C-1). As you unfold your leg try to extend your calf up over your thigh (Fig. 7C-2). Hold leg under knee so you don't pull calf in. The area behind the knees is often tight. Don't try for a "straight" leg, just gently yield where you are.

8. Pelvis and Legs

The relationship of the pelvis to the legs and to the rest of the spine must be free to move in harmony with the unity of the mechanism. If the lower back or the hip sockets are held, the freedom set up by the reflexes in the head cannot reverberate throughout the body. This next set of processes is designed to bring awareness to these very specific spots of over-contraction.

In America, lower back trouble plagues more people than any other illness. There are, of course, many reasons for this. One reason is that most people do not and cannot allow movement to take place in the hip socket, a ball and socket joint, that is so designed for movement. Instead they move from the lower back, which is not designed as a locomotor. As a consequence, weight collects in the inactive hip area. One must learn to stop pulling the lower back and to find, free, and use the hip sockets.

Process 8A: Relationship of Pelvis

Sit back on your feet. As you breathe out, come forward with the pubic bone as far as you can (Fig. 8A-1). Pelvic crest goes back and up, as pubic bone comes more forward. Keep knees together. Do not arch back. Push forward below and behind your buttocks, but don't tighten to do it. Freedom in the neck leads. If you cannot sit on your feet comfortably you may do it lying down with the legs bent. *Figure 8A-2 is incorrect because the lower back is arched.*

Fig. 8A-1	Fig. 8A-2

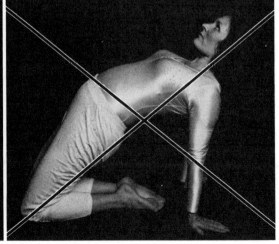

Process 8B: To Find Hip Sockets

1.   Lie on the floor on your back, knees bent, arms horizontal by sides (Fig. 8B-1).

Fig. 8B-1

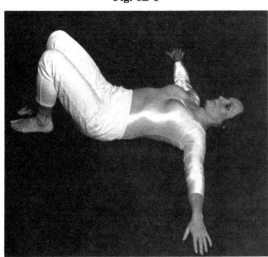

2. Straighten one leg by lengthening through the calf and heel (Fig. 8B-2).

3. Return by allowing the knee to go to the ceiling. Other leg.

4. Breathe in—on out breath, raise pubic bone and then return to the floor (Fig. 8B-3).

5. Walk feet around to left side of your body with small steps. Do not move pelvis (Fig. 8B-4). Return to center. Other side.

Fig. 8B-2

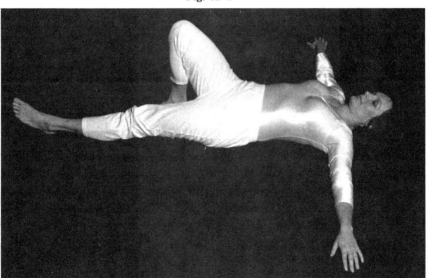

Fig. 8B-3

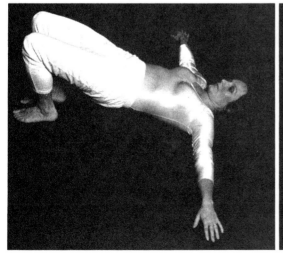

Fig. 8B-4

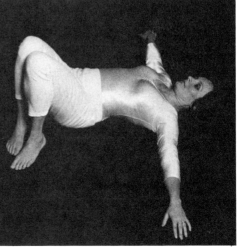

6.   Walk shoulders to right side of your body (Fig. 8B-5). Return to center. Other side. Keep waist on the floor and knees vertical to the floor.

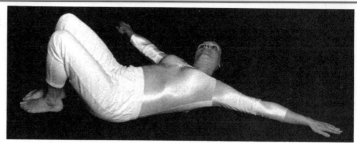

Fig. 8B-5

Process 8C: To Loosen Hip Sockets

1.   Sit on the floor cross-legged (Fig. 8C-1). Now pick your buttocks off the floor. Keep heels pushing forward. Put your hands in front of your knees to keep them from coming forward.

2.   Pull pubic bone forward, turn legs in socket (Fig. 8C-2).

Fig. 8C-1

Fig. 8C-2

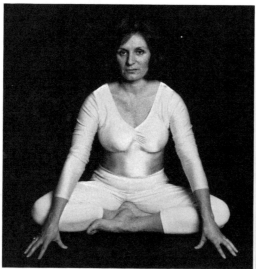
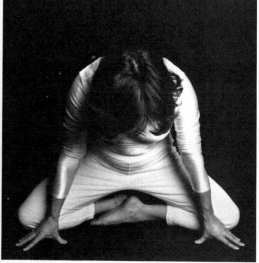

Process 8D: Lying down to release hips

1.   Lie on your stomach on the floor, arms out, legs straight (Fig. 8D-1).

2.   Bend right knee and bring it up to right shoulder, keeping your knee on the floor (Fig. 8D-2). Allow hip socket to release down toward outstretched knee (Fig. 8D-3) and allow pubic bone to fall to the floor as pelvic crest comes back and up and breathe.

3.   Straighten the leg (Fig. 8D-4).

4.   Return and do other leg.

Fig. 8D-1   Fig. 8D-2

Fig. 8D-3   Fig. 8D-4

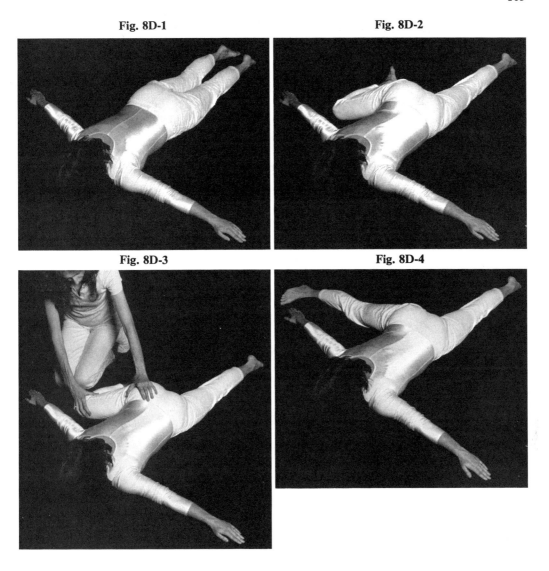

Process 8E: Deep Hip Sockets Release

1.   Lie on your stomach on the floor. Knees are bent and split apart, and soles of your feet are together, chest on the floor. Rest head (Fig. 8E-1).

Fig. 8E-1   Fig. 8E-2

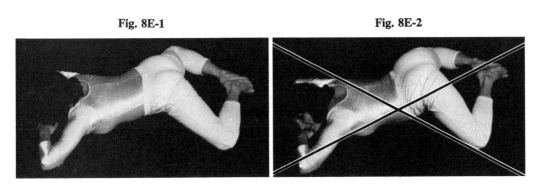

2. On out breath, turn bottom of pelvis under, not in *lower back*, but in socket. Stay here and breathe. Allow gravity to take your pubic bone to the floor as knees go out away from each other. If this is not too uncomfortable, for more stretch, bring one knee up to shoulder and then the other. Don't arch the lower back (Fig. 8E-2). You may put pads under your knees for comfort.

Process 8F: Stretch Top Thigh

Often a tight hip socket is coupled with a tight top front thigh. To extend heels down, we don't need to push the seat back.

1. Lie on your side, knees bent (Fig. 8F-1).
2. Bend top leg forward to chest, then extend it out through heel (Fig. 8F-2).
3. Hold top of the pelvic crest up and back. Push forward under buttocks as leg goes down (Fig. 8F-3).
4. Have a partner pull the heel out and pull the crest back (Fig. 8F-4).

Fig. 8F-1

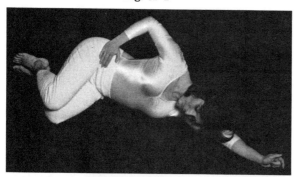

Fig. 8F-2

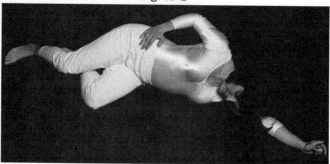

Fig. 8F-3

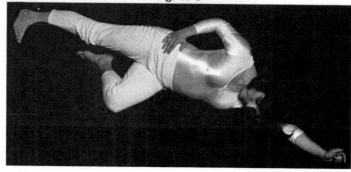

Fig. 8F-4

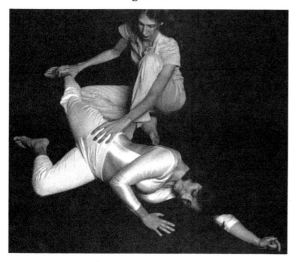

Fig. 8G

Process 8G: Back to Wall

1. Stand against a wall with heels touching it, feet parallel.
2. Allow knees to bend forward until your lower back touches the wall. As you get up allow your back to come back and up against the wall. Free your heels into the floor as your head leads

Fig. 8H-1   Fig. 8H-2

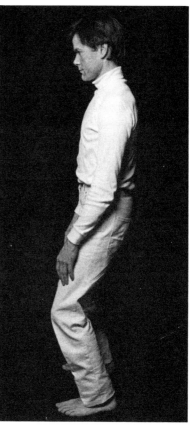

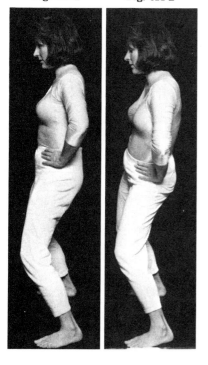

up. This process is not to take the curves out of your back but to stimulate the spiralic support muscles so the hips can be free (Fig. 8G). Repeat.

Process 8H: Figure Eight

Stand with legs apart. Make a figure eight with your pelvis—front, side, back, side (Figs. 8H-1, 2). As they go to the side don't cut the corners. Large curves increase rotational possibilities. To do this you must open in front hips and use rotators in back. This loosens the hip socket.

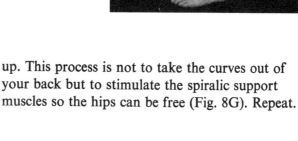

Fig. 8I-1

Fig. 8I-2

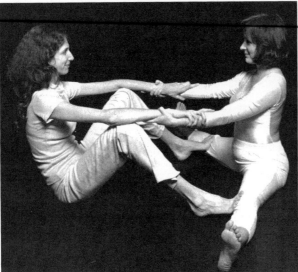

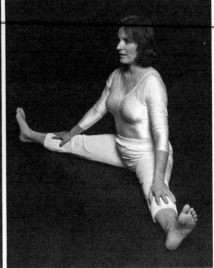

Fig. 8I-3

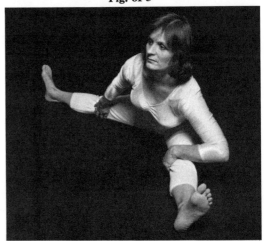

Process 8I: Rotation in Hip Socket (Beginner)

1.   Helper sits and holds your hands and pushes your knees back with her feet (Fig. 8I-1).

2.   Move your torso in a small circle and spiral out to a bigger circle. Push out through heels (Figs. 8I-2–5).

Fig. 8I-4

Fig. 8I-5

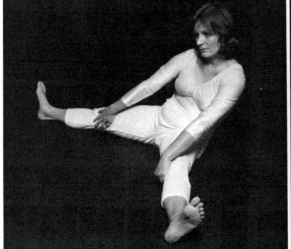

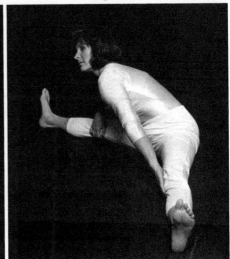

Process 8J: Rotation in hip socket (Intermediate)

1. Sit with legs open on floor, feet flexed.
2. Lift torso, then stretch chest to floor, with hands on the floor (Fig. 8J-1).
3. Come up and bring legs together (Fig. 8J-2).
4. Push up through heels and bring feet overhead (Fig. 8J-3).
5. Open legs wide and roll down to starting position (Fig. 8J-4).

Fig. 8J-1

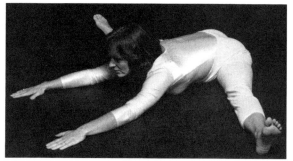

Fig. 8J-2

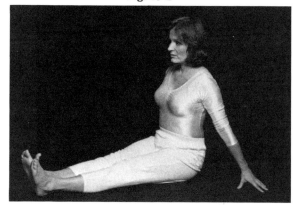

Fig. 8J-3

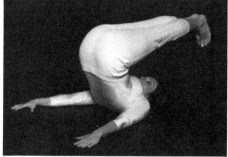

Figl 8J-4

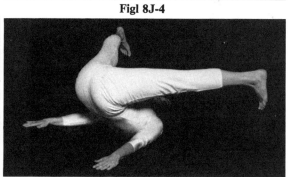

Fig. 8K-1

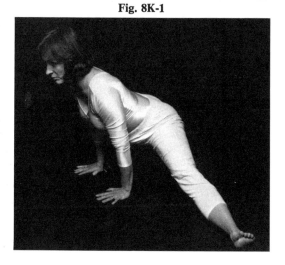

Process 8K: Rotation in Hip Socket (Advanced)

1. Sit legs apart on floor. Arms in front of you, elbows on the floor. Walk hands and reach until buttocks lift up (Fig. 8K-1).

168

Fig. 8K-2

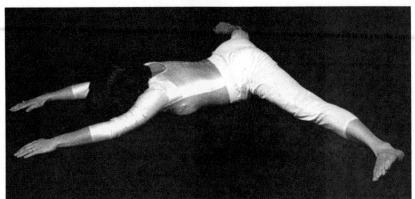

Fig. 8K-3

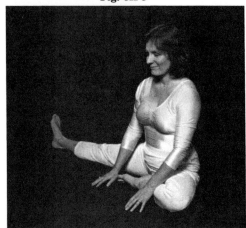

2. Keep going forward and lie on stomach (pubic bone leads, not pelvic crest) (Fig. 8K-2).

3. Walk arms in and return by pushing buttocks down.

4. Try it with one leg bent (Figs. 8K-3-4). Do not arch back! (Fig. 8K-5).

Fig. 8K-4

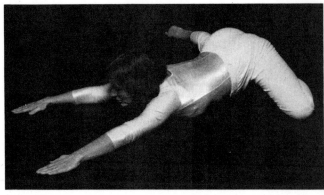

Fig. 8K-5

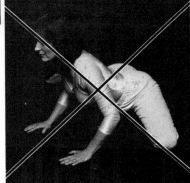

9. Propulsion

Process 9A: Rolling

1. Sit with legs crossed, reaching arms forward on the floor.

Fig. 9A-1

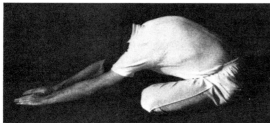

Fig. 9A-2

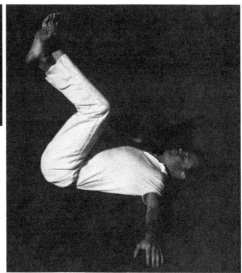

2.   Roll onto your back as hands circle out to the sides along the floor. Return same path. Roll back and forth (Figs. 9A-1–3). If you cannot sit cross-legged, a squatting position is fine. Tuck head and roll up and down.

Fig. 9A-3

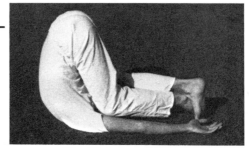

Process 9B: Swing Legs

1.   Begin sitting. Bend legs to one side (Fig. 9B-1).

Fig. 9B-1

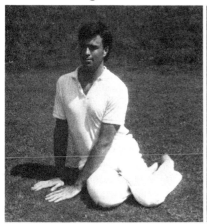

Fig. 9B-2

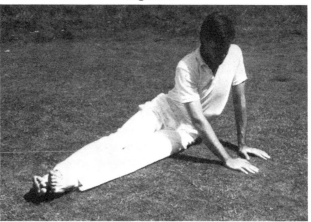

Fig. 9B-3

Fig. 9B-4

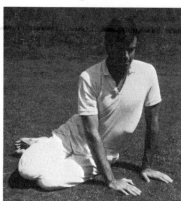

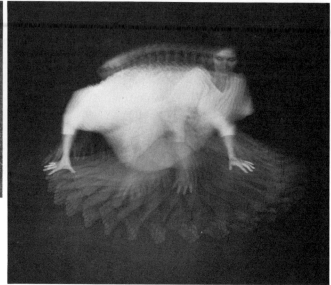

2.   Then unfold legs and swing them halfway around in front of you (Fig. 9B-2) and bend to the other side (Fig. 9B-3). Don't bend legs too soon.

3.   Advanced–try to swing legs all the way around. Keep head and torso facing the same direction—front. Move arms as needed. Other side. In motion, Figure 9B-4.

Process 9C: Diagonal Reach Back

1.   Begin sitting with buttocks on heels. Reach diagonally back to right side, placing hands on the floor and bending elbows (Fig. 9C-1).

2.   Repeat to left side (Fig. 9C-2).

Fig. 9C-1

Fig. 9C-2

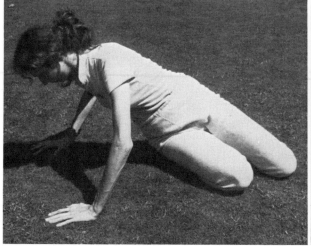

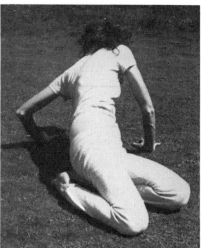

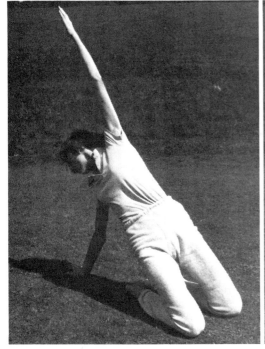

Fig. 9C-3

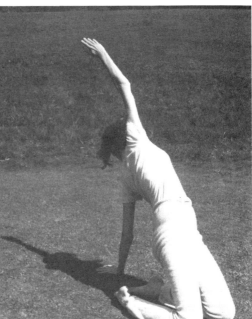

Fig. 9C-4

Fig. 9D-1

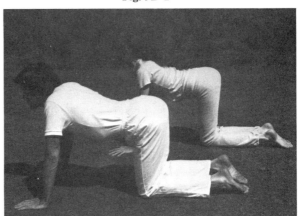

3.   Reach diagonally back to the right side, put right hand on the floor, and lift pelvis (Fig. 9C-3).

4.   Reach to left high diagonal (Fig. 9C-4).

Process 9D: On Hands and Knees

1.   On the floor on your hands and knees, breathe in.

2.   On out breath arch back (Fig. 9D-1).

3.   Return and breathe in.

4.   Breathe out and hump back up (Fig. 9D-2).

Fig. 9D-2

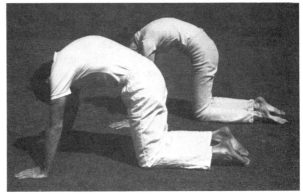

172

Fig. 9D-3

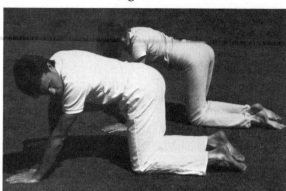

5. Return and breathe in.
6. Look over right shoulder at right hip. Breathe out.
7. Return and breathe in.
8. Look over left shoulder at left hip and breathe out (Fig. 9D-3).
9. Breathe in and on out breath extend right arm and left leg (Fig. 9D-4).

Fig. 9D-4

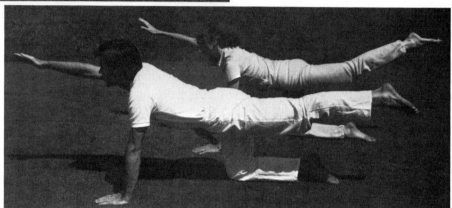

Fig. 9D-5

10. Breathe in and on out breath bring right elbow and left knee together (Fig. 9D-5).
11. Breathe in and extend same as 9 (Fig. 9D-6).

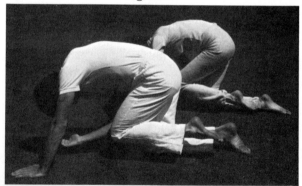

Fig. 9D-6

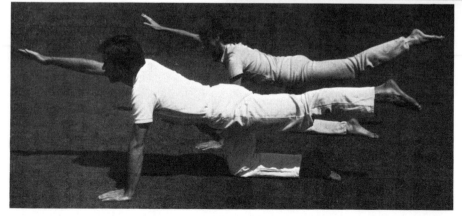

Fig. 9D-7

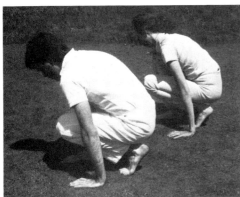

12. Now walk through your arms (Fig. 9D-7) so legs are straight in front of you.

13. Sit for one second (Fig. 9D-8) and return back walking through legs (Fig. 9D-9). Don't lift up in shoulders to do it. The problem is the stretch down the back of your leg. (Don't avoid it.) Yield. Keep legs in a parallel, don't let them pull together.

Fig. 9D-8

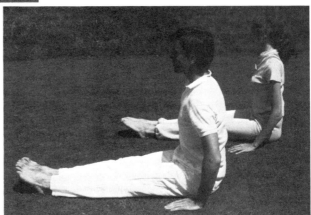

Fig. 9D-9

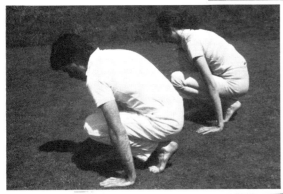

14. Variation: Repeat steps 1–9 (Fig. 9D-10).

Fig. 9D-10

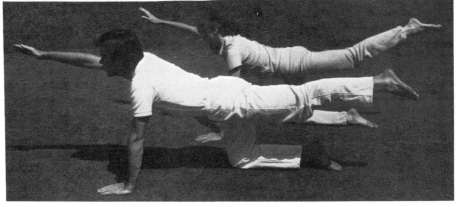

Fig. 9D-11

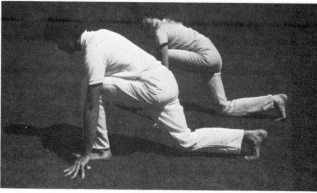

Fig. 9D-12

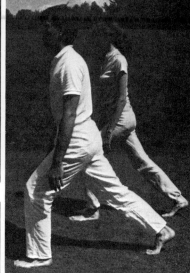

Fig. 9D-13

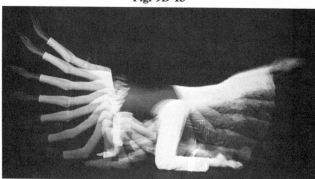

15.   Breathe in and on out breath return right hand to floor as left foot steps through arms to walk forward (Fig. 9D-11). As you walk do not let buttocks fall back (Fig. 9D-12). Repeat other side. In motion, Fig. 9D-13.

Process 9E: Across the Floor

1.   Stand on your hands and knees, pelvis over knees (Fig. 9E-1).
2.   Lift left elbow and left knee. Extend both to straight (Fig. 9E-2).
3.   Turn until you sit and spiral left elbow and left knee in (Fig. 9E-3).
4.   Pick up right elbow and right knee (Fig. 9E-4).

Fig. 9E-1   Fig. 9E-2

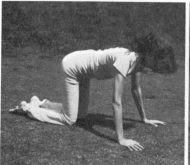
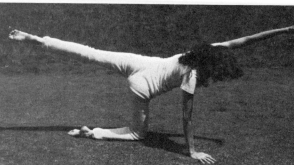

175

Fig. 9E-3   Fig. 9E-4

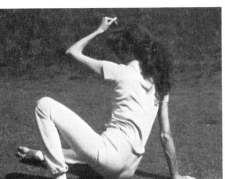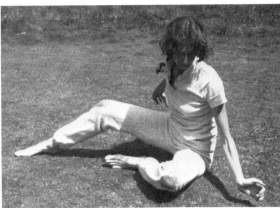

Fig. 9E-5

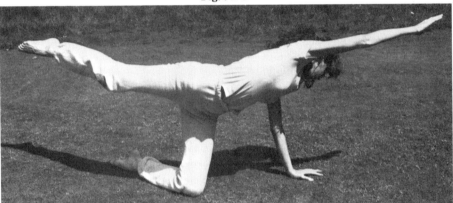

Fig. 9E-6

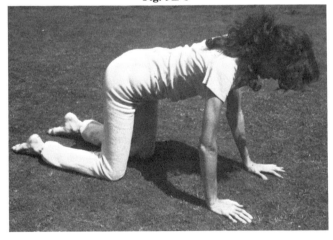

5. Extend them to straight (Fig. 9E-5) and spiral them in as you continue to roll over like a barrel (Fig. 9E-6). Both knee and elbow land at the same time. Back stays in one line. When turning, don't lift shoulders. Lift hand and foot together. Do not arch back.

Don't manipulate yourself—let things happen.

10. Spiral in Leg

Process 10A: Knee Down-heel Up

If the plantaurus muscle (the muscle on the outside of your calf) is tight, it will pull your knee in toward center and pull your foot out and away from center. You want to lengthen the outside lower leg to prevent this.

1.   To correct this sit on the floor. Make the knee the center of a cone-shaped circle and move your *heel* in a circle at the bottom of this cone shape. This loosens your knee joint.

Fig. 10A-1

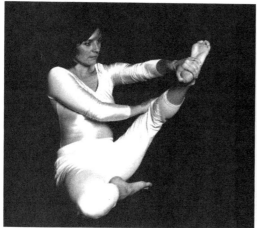

Fig. 10A-2

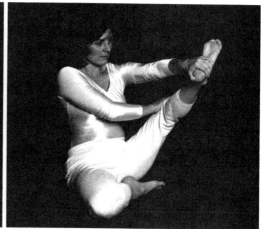

Fig. 10A-3

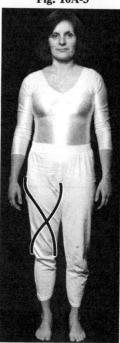

2.   Take your left foot with your left hand and put your right hand on the inside of your left knee (do not wrap it around). Keep your left leg in front of your nose, not to the side (Fig. 10A-1).

3.   Push your knee to the floor and pull your heel to the ceiling (Fig. 10A-2). Do not twist the foot. Eventually you straighten the leg but not by locking the knee and rotating it inward. When doing knee down-heel up make sure knee is turned very far back. As you push out through the heel don't internally rotate the thigh. When doing knee down-heel up feel the opposite side of body (of leg that's working) pulling forward to the leg. Don't sit back. This process creates muscle balance, not power.

The diagonal pulls in the thigh are the inside back knee connecting to the outside front thigh, and a line from the inside back thigh to outside front knee (Fig. 10A-3). Try to lengthen the inside of the thigh as much as the outside.

Process 10B: Parallel Calf Stretch

1.   Sit on the floor on the front of your pelvic bones, bending your knees. Hold the balls of your feet from the side (Fig. 10B-1). Pull toes toward you. Let your feet totally relax. Toes are together. Heels are apart. Don't bend the metatarsal joint, keeping your feet flat as if they were on a floor. Knees are apart. Breathe in and bring legs (bend knees) to chest.

2.   *Keep chest on thighs.* Breathe out. Push through heels. Brace knees out and keep toes together and heels apart (Fig. 10B-2). Only go as far as you can go with your chest on your thighs. Otherwise you avoid the stretch (Fig. 10B-3). Stay there and breathe. Sits bones back and heels forward. To continue the stretch in the back, it is important not to raise the shoulders, but to allow the width in the back. To come up, use arms to bring feet up, not leg muscles, because if you use leg muscles you contract them and have to start with shorter muscles. This process dissolves excess yang or will put in needed yang to lower body. It is good for the bladder meridian, and knee and lower back pain. In motion, Figure 10B-4.

Fig. 10B-1   Fig. 10B-2

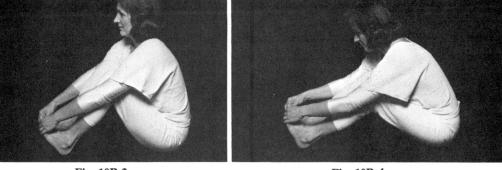

Fig. 10B-3   Fig. 10B-4

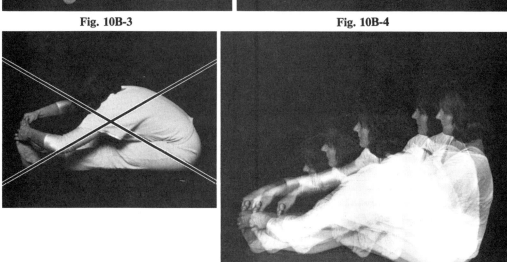

Process 10C: Walk Tight Rope

Many calves tend to push out to the side. (See Chapter 4, Fig. 7). This does not support correct rotation in the leg.

To correct this:

1.   Hold knees out apart with a fist. This gets inside calf muscles to pull toward center instead of toward the outside. Rotate your calves out against the inward pull of the thigh. Pretend you are walking a tightrope, on one straight line (Fig. 10C-1). Allow heel to lengthen (stretch calf) before you step. Good for imbalance in kidney, liver or spleen meridians and for straightening crooked legs.

2.   Try two fists (Fig. 10C-2).

Fig. 10C-1 **Fig. 10C-2**

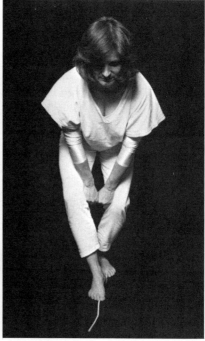

11.   Feet

Process 11A: The Diagonal Pulls

The diagonal pulls in the foot (see Fig. 11A): these pulls should be equal for a stable base. Try to stand with these diagonals in mind, with no "gripping" in the toes or foot and realize that you are being supported by the earth.

Fig. 11A

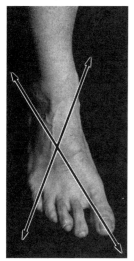

Process 11B: Stretch Top Foot

If there is tightness on the top of the foot: sit on the floor with the knees bent. Put the top of the foot under a radiator or someone's hands, then slowly straighten the legs (Fig. 11B).

Process 11C: Foot Spines

The bottom of the foot has two arches or spines: one lengthwise and one widthwise (Fig. 11C). Try to fold both sides of the foot around the arch. This knits the bottom of the foot together.

Fig. 11B

Fig. 11C

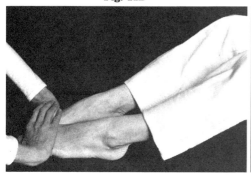

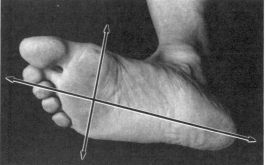

Process 11D: Toe Meridians

Note on callouses: why do some people get callouses and others don't? And some in one place and some in another place? When excesses of certain foods or chemicals

Fig. 11D

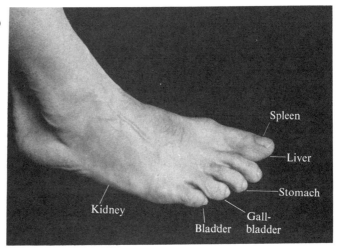

are eaten the body cannot process them so it eliminates them. One way is through the skin. Excesses usually come out around an energy center or acupuncture point. Excess proteins and fats often discharge through the feet, something like a little volcano or callous. These may be rubbed off with a pumice stone (available in natural food stores). Once a more balanced diet is adapted they will not reappear.

The foot, in addition to other parts of the body, contains reflex points for the whole body. The summer of 1973 I taught shiatsu massage at a dance camp in New York. One man, literally dragged by his wife, came to class. When we worked on the feet, I pointed out that the base of the big toe was a reflex point for the head. When pressed, it may relieve all headaches, even migraines. He perked up because he suffered this ailment. He missed the next class because of an airplane trip to San Francisco. While he was on the plane he felt a migraine coming on. To his dismay he remembered his pills were packed away in his luggage. When he could bear the pain no more, he said, "What the heck," and took off his shoe and sock in the first class section of the plane and rubbed the base of his big toe until the pain subsided.

12. Purification

These sequences are used to release toxins, increase blood flow and circulation, and wake up the being. They should be done with a big out breath. They can be used to develop the hara (below navel, second chakra). To do this keep energy awareness 1) on the big toe; 2) on inside knee; 3) on hara; and 4) on keeping chin in.

Process 12A: Up and Down

1.   Start hands and feet on floor, buttocks in the air (Fig. 12A-1).
2.   Jump so that hips, toes, and hands are on the floor with open legs (Fig. 12A-2). Return to step 1. Repeat 10 times fast. Relax.

Fig. 12A-1

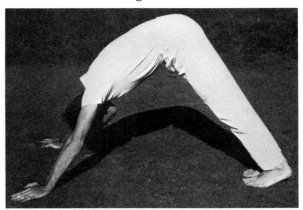

Fig. 12A-2

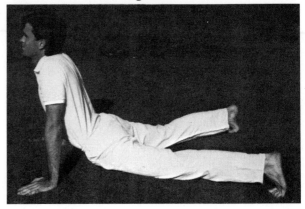

Process 12B: Twist Side to Side

1. Start hands under arms, legs open 45 degrees and standing on toes (Fig. 12B-1).
2. Exhale and jump and twist head to look at left heel (Fig. 12B-2). Both heels to floor.
3. Return center (Fig. 12B-3).
4. Other side (Figs. 12B-4 and 5). Repeat 10 times fast and relax.

Fig. 12B-1

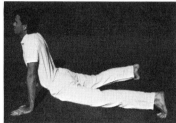

Fig. 12B-2

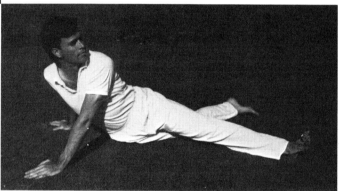

Fig. 12B-3

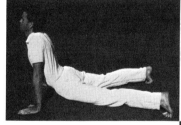

Fig. 12B-4

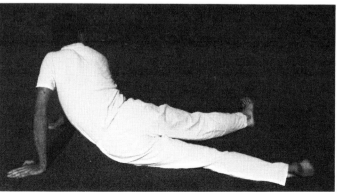

Fig. 12B-5

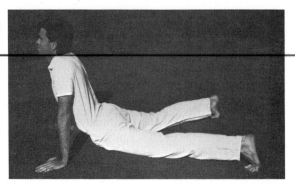

Fig. 12B-5

Process 12C: Diagonal Swing

1. Sit on floor, legs open, left arm behind you (Fig. 12C-1).
2. Lift hips and swing left arm across body to the high right corner (Figs. 12C-2 and 3).

Fig. 12C-1

Fig. 12C-2

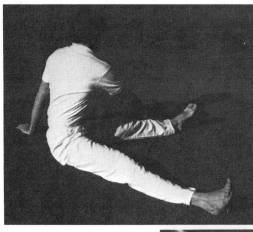

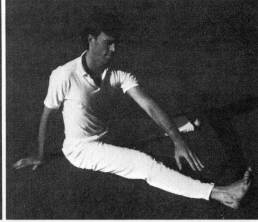

Fig. 12C-3

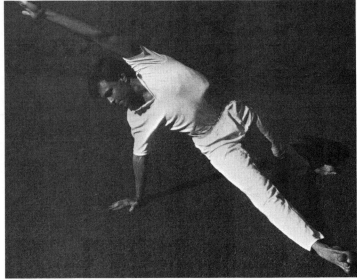

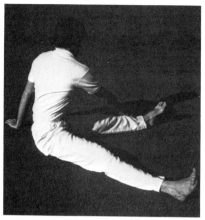

Fig. 12C-4

3. Return (Fig. 12C-4). Other side, 10 times fast.

Process 12D: Hip Twist

1. Begin on knees and forearms (Fig. 12D-1).
2. Take hips to right side (Fig. 12D-2).
3. Return center (Fig. 12D-3).
4. Hips to left (Fig. 12D-4).
5. Return center (Fig. 12D-5). Ten times fast.

Fig. 12D-1

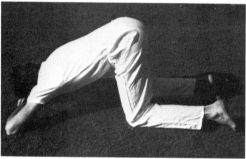

Fig. 12D-2

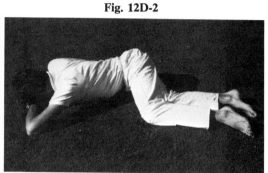

Fig. 12D-3

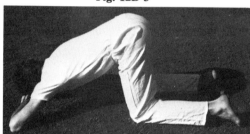

Fig. 12D-4

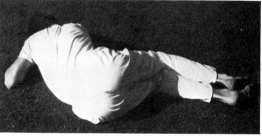

Fig. 12D-5

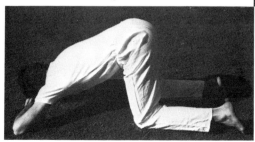

Process 12E: Around the Clock

This process is good for the intestines.
1. Begin standing, arms overhead (Fig. 12E-1).
2. Reach out through hands, around the clock on out breath. 12 o'clock, 11 o'clock, 10 o'clock, and so on. (Figs. 12E-2–5).

Fig. 12E-1

Fig. 12E-2

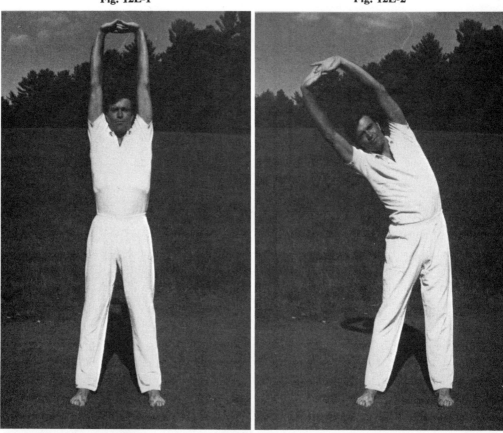

Fig. 12E-3

Fig. 12E-4

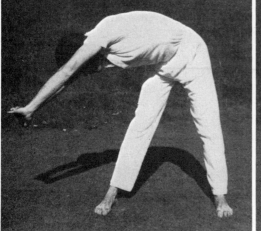
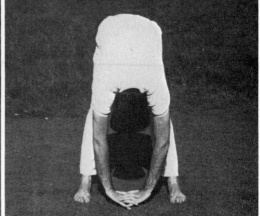

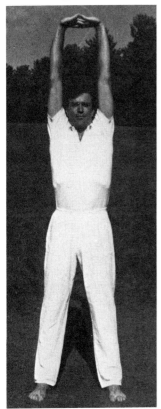

Fig. 12E-5

3. Repeat other direction.

Process 12F: Jogging

Once I was driving with my mother near the ocean. We passed a jogger and she said to me, "I've never seen a jogger with a happy face." Ideally, it is great to be out-side in fresh air, to be moving through space, to see the scenery move by, to feel the elements (the cold, the sun or rain). But many joggers do not notice these.

A few pointers:

1. Do not pull your head back and down as many runners do.

2. Run with as little tension all over as possible (watch shoulders).

3. Run on grass when possible.

4. Do not pull lower leg up after you step on it. This increases calf tension (Illus. 4).

Illus. 4

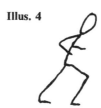

5. Since jogging is done in the same plane of movement, I recommend spiral sequences before or after. This helps develop muscle fibers in a more rounded fashion. If the body is used correctly the spiralic nature of the muscle will automatically be stimulated.

13. Partners

A child asked his grandfather, "What is the difference between heaven and hell?" The grandfather answered, "There is a big room. It is filled with hungry people and they have plenty of food in their bowls on the table. The problem is that they have very long spoons and cannot get them to their mouths. This is hell. There is a second room exactly like the first. But in this room the people are using the long spoons to feed each other. This is heaven."

Process 13A: Minimal Energy

Let all energy go and fall to the floor. No energy. Then feel energy in all parts. Move with minimal energy but feel it all. Use *least* to move. Finally get up using minimal energy.

Take a partner. Stand palms to palms. Push each other with minimal weight and energy. Stand with pelvis vertical, feet planted on floor and top of the back leaning slightly forward. Push with whole body, not just arms (Fig. 13A).

Fig. 13A

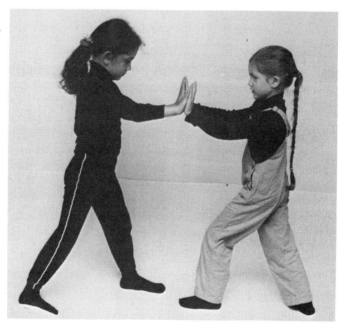

Process 13B: For Opening Across Chest

Have one person on each side of your shoulders (Fig. 13B). Let arms relax down.

Fig. 13B

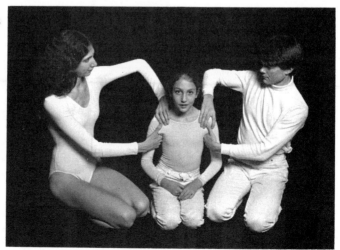

The helpers will pull the shoulder girdle down and out. Shoulders yield outward and upper arms widen.

Process 13C: Freeing Joints

Brace foot on one part and gently pull to free a joint.
   1.   To free hip sockets: brace foot on hip crest and gently lean back, holding heel (Fig. 13C-1).
   2.   To free arm: hold wrist and pull arm. Brace foot on ribs (Fig. 13C-2).

Fig. 13C-1

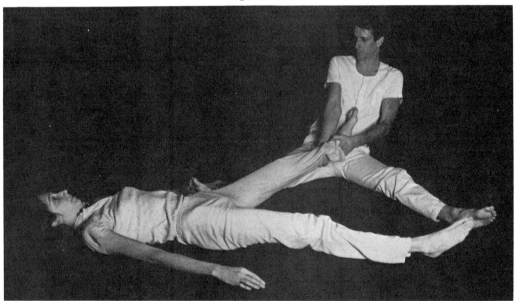

Fig. 13C-2

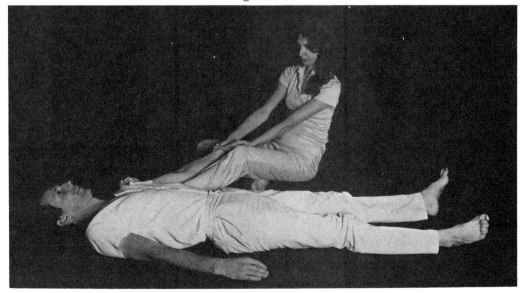

Fig. 13C-3

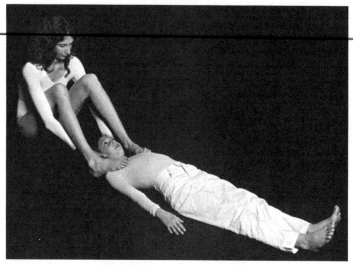

Fig. 13C-4

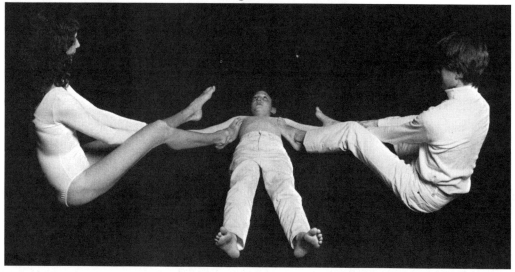

3. To stretch neck: brace feet on shoulders and *gently* take head forward and up (Fig. 13C-3).

4. One person lies down, five people pull. Two pull hands and two pull feet and one holds head gently (Fig. 13C-4) (minus 3 people).

Process 13D: Stretch Backs

1. One person stands on knees, arms overhead. Partner stands and holds arms over head (Fig. 13D-1).

2. Put buttocks on upper back and pull arms up and out as you push forward between shoulder blades (Figs. 13D-2 and 3). We do not push forward in the lower back because on most people it is already over-arched.

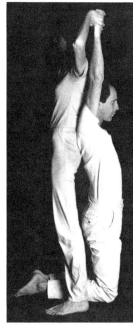

Fig. 13D-1

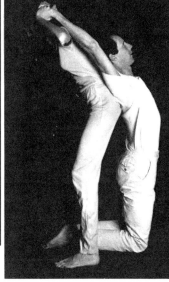

Fig. 13D-2

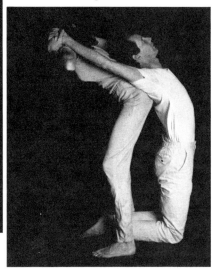

Fig. 13D-3

Process 13E: Spiral Arm and Leg

1.   Partner lies on right side. Helper sits on the floor and holds right ankle and left wrist and puts one foot on partner's sacrum, not in lumbar region (Fig. 13E-1).

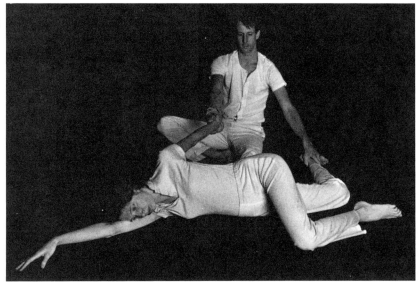

Fig. 13E-1

190

2. As he breathes out, pull ankle and wrist, stretch upper and lower back evenly (Figs. 13E-2 and 3).

Fig. 13E-2

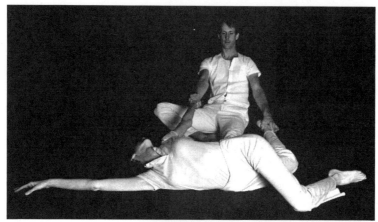

Fig. 13E-3

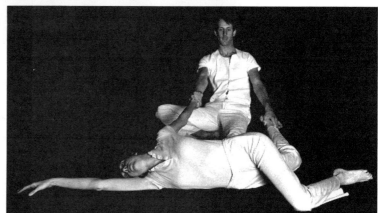

Process 13F: Back to Back

1. Interlock arms and sit back to back.
2. Both partners circle torso around. One partner leans forward while the other

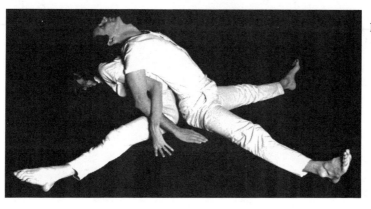

Fig. 13F-1

leans back to give stretch (Figs. 13F-1–4).

3.   Circle other way.

4.   One partner lies on the other partner's back (Figs. 13F-5 and 6).

Fig. 13F-2

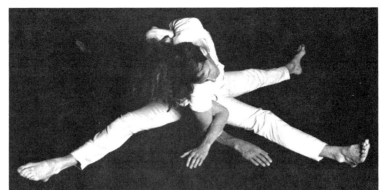

Fig. 13F-3

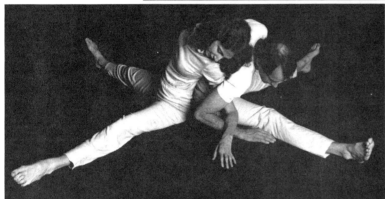

Fig. 13F-4

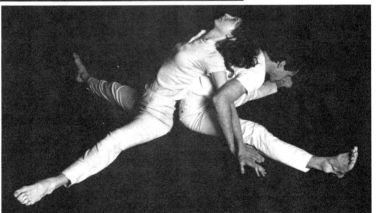

Fig. 13F-5

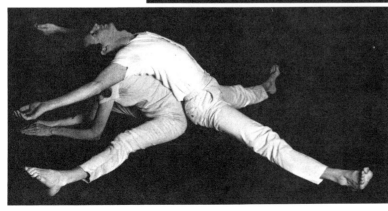

Fig. 13F-6

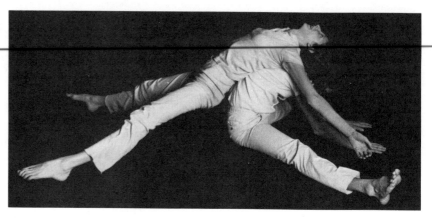

Process 13G: Circle Torso

Sit on the floor with legs open, hold arms and circle torsos around (Figs. 13G-1–4).

Fig. 13G-1

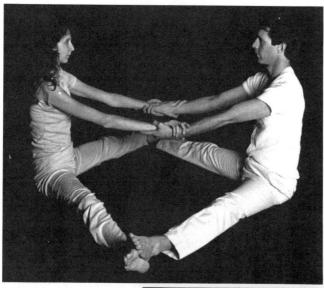

Fig. 13G-2

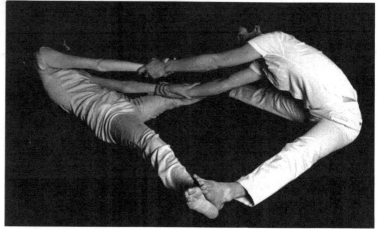

193

Fig. 13G-3

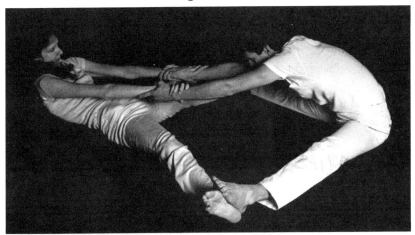

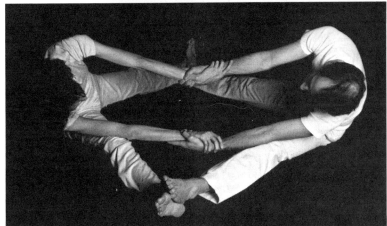

Fig. 13G-4

Fig. 13H

Process 13H: Walk on Thighs

Partner sits on heels, arms behind buttocks. Helper puts hands on shoulders, feet on thighs and walks up and down thighs. Good for overeating and stomach (Fig. 13H).

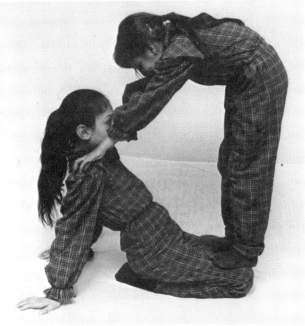

194

Fig. 13I-1

Fig. 13I-2

Fig. 13I-3

Fig. 13I-4

Fig. 13I-5

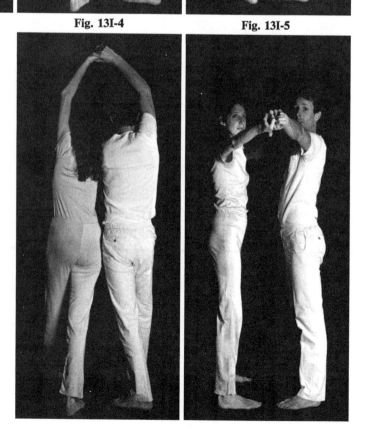

Process 13I: Turn Around Arms

1. Stand facing partner (Fig. 13I-1), arms out to the side parallel to floor.
2. On out breath reach one arm down and one arm over head (Fig. 13I-2).
3. Reach until the arms are again parallel to the floor with the upper body twisted (Fig. 13I-3). Move the feet on the floor as little as possible.
4. Return the way you came (Fig. 13I-4).
5. Do other side (Fig. 13I-5). The stretch for the arms is good for the chest and lungs.

Process 13J: Arm Stretch

Both partners stand so that torso is gradually perpendicular to legs. Put arms on partner's upper back (Figs. 13J-1–3). As you breathe out, give slight down push on upper back to get stretch under armpit (Fig. 13J-4). Change arm positions to be on the inside. Good for lung and heart meridians.

Fig. 13J-1

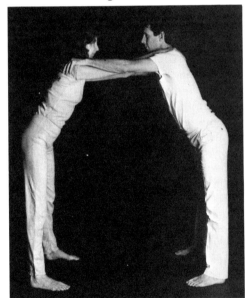

Fig. 13J-2

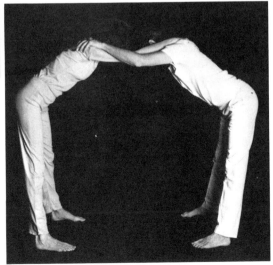

196

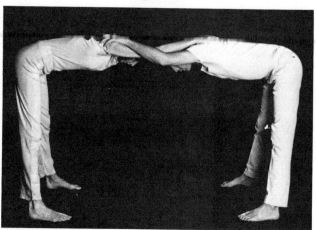

Fig. 13J-3

Fig. 13J-4

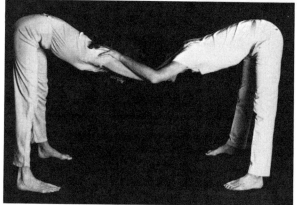

Process 13K: Balance

Hold each other's arms. Both lean slightly back. Free head forward and up and send knees forward and heels down. Keep the spatial tension from pubic bone to head. Don't break in the waist (Figs. 13K-1–5).

Fig. 13K-1

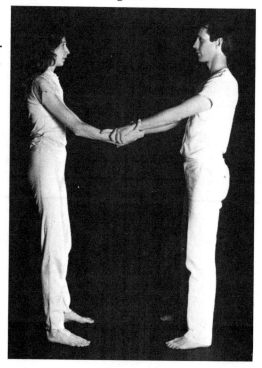

197

Fig. 13K-2

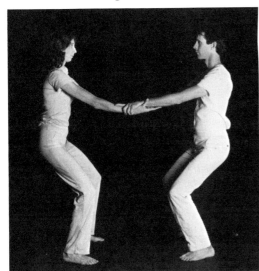

Fig. 13K-3

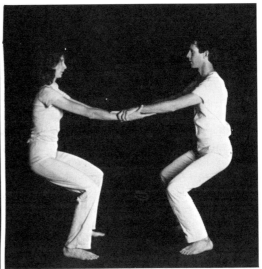

Fig. 13K-4

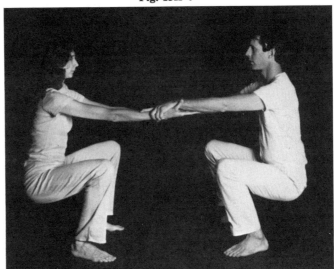

Fig. 13K-5

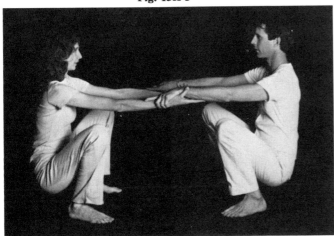

Process 13L: Dynamic Balance

Hold hands or wrists, feet together (Fig. 13L-1). One sits down while the other balances standing up. Pull each other up and down (Figs. 13L-2–9). As you stand push heels down, head leads up. Lower back leads back. Arms straight. Buttocks go as far away from feet as possible. In motion, Figure 13L-10.

Fig. 13L-1

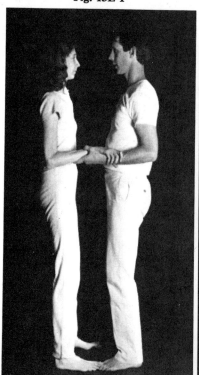

Fig. 13L-2

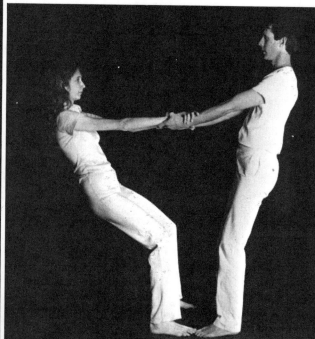

Fig. 13L-3

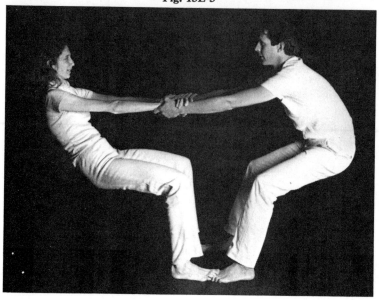

Fig. 13L-4

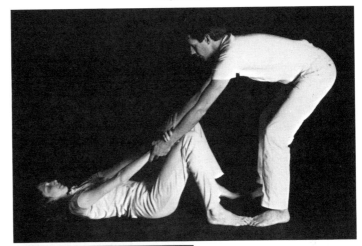

Fig. 13L-5

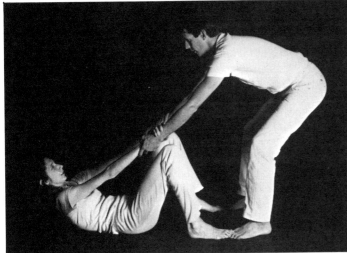

Fig. 13L-6

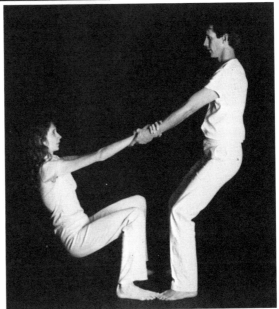

200

Fig. 13L-7

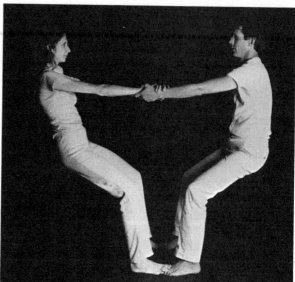

Fig. 13L-8

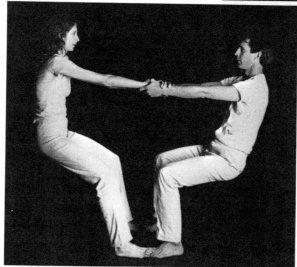

Fig. 13L-9

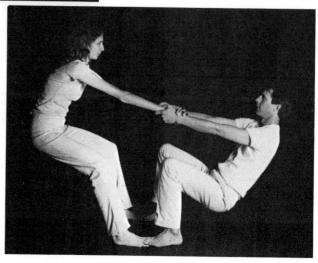

Fig. 13L-10

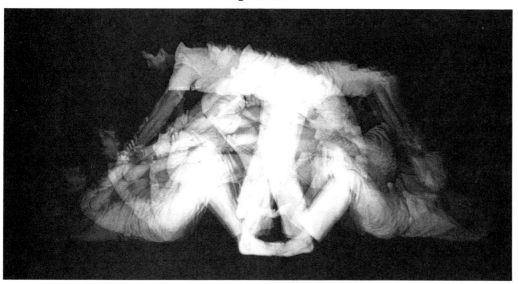

14. To Relax

Process 14A: Pick Up Parts

Lie on the floor on your back—relax, no work. One partner picks up parts of body and the other person just lets go (Figs. 14A-1–3). Notice your tension.

Fig. 14A-1

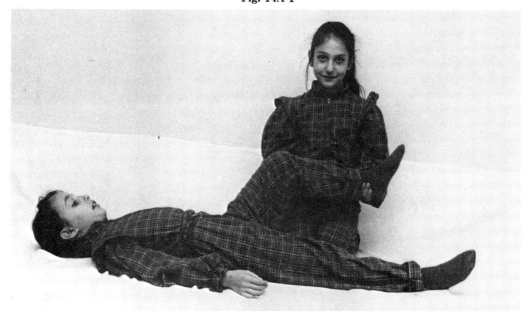

Fig. 14A-2

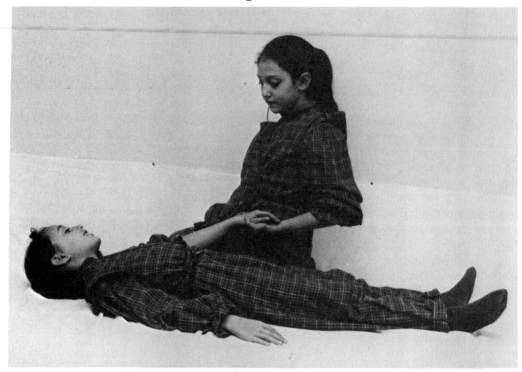

Fig. 14A-3

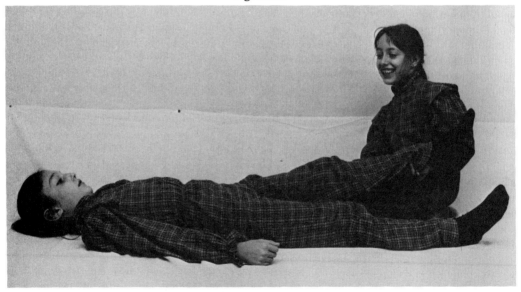

Process 14B: Water Bag

Push flexed feet back and forth like a water bag (Fig. 14B).

Fig. 14B

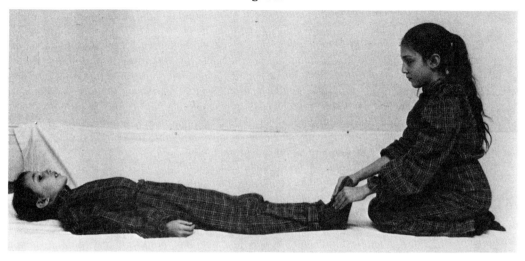

Process 14C: Swing Legs

Swing legs side to side (Fig. 14C).

Fig. 14C

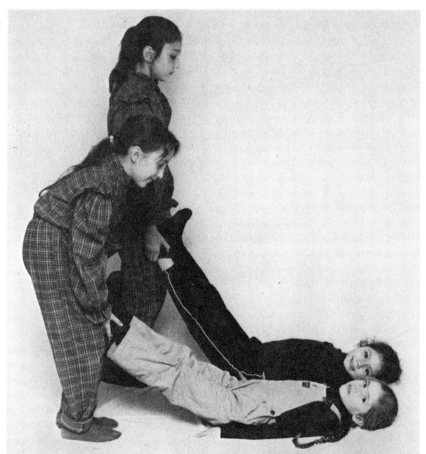

204

Process 14D: Shake Knee

Lie on stomach and bend leg. Partner shakes knee up and down (Fig. 14D).

Fig. 14D

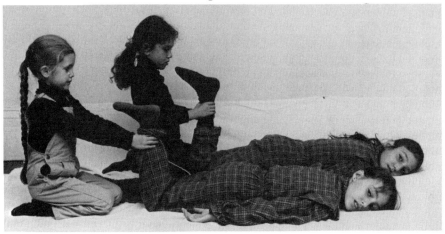

Process 14E: Release Legs

Lie on stomach. Partner holds legs up and pushes coccyx forward (Fig. 14E). Meditative quality leads to the divine.

Fig. 14E

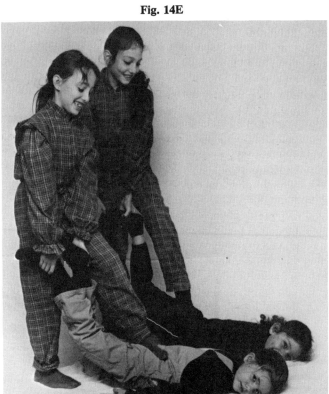

In Closing

Throughout the ages the traditional condemns the modern ways. Progress, technology and experiments fascinate the brain. But as we have seen, yang at the extreme will change to yin. It is wonderful to move ahead with "progress" if the whole self —mental, physical and spiritual—can keep up with the pace. Motion and stillness must balance.

If we don't build the quiet breathing space into our lives consciously, stops will come unconsciously through sickness or change. There is space in every moment for choice. But because the decision must harmonize with the existing whole, there seems to be no choice.

We all look at each other and think, "I know the way and he doesn't," or "He knows the way and I don't." Dwelling on this only separates. We each have our own part. Books or teachers may inspire or provoke, but only you are responsible for your actions. There are no victims.

In changing your life don't be afraid to ask questions or make mistakes. They are better than being stuck. You can only pick your path by walking on it. Your journey on the spiral of life progresses to your delight and takes a sharp curve when you least expect it. If I have stepped on anyone's toes, I hope it is only enough to stimulate, but not to hurt.

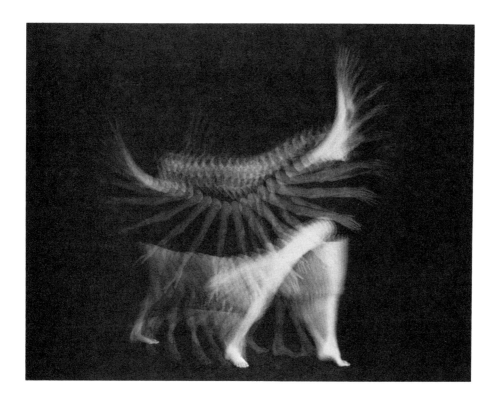

Notes

Chapter 1

[1]"Voluntary Musculature in the Human Body" p. 8.

[2]*The Book of Macrobiotics*, p. 9.

[3]*The Power of Limits* contains elaborate explanations of these principles.

[4]*Power of Limits*, p. 28.

[5]*Behold Man*, p. 229.

[6]Adapted from Gorman, *The Body Moveable*.

[7]*The Body Moveable*, Volume I, p. 50.

[8]Figures adapted from *The Body Moveable*, Illus. 14, 15, 18, 20, 25, 29, 33, 37, 40, 43.

[9]"Voluntary Musculature in the Human Body," quoting *Human Potential*, Vol. I, No. 2, 1968.

[10]"Voluntary Musculature in the Human Body," p. 7.

[11]Some material from this section was extrapolated from "The Evolution of the Living Body" series by David Gorman.

[12]*The Way of Life*, p. 94.

[13]*The Way of Life*, p. 94.

[14]*Gospel According to Thomas*, p. 3.

[15]*The Way of Life*, p. 95.

[16]*The Way of Life*, p. 95.

Chapter 2

[1]*Body Awareness in Action*, p. 159.

[2]*The Book of Dance*, p. 26.

[3]*Balletomania Then and Now*, p. 59.

[4]*An Introduction to the Teachings of Bhagwan Shree Rajneesh—Dance*

[5]*The Dance Through the Ages*, p. 52, quote by L.S. Ramaswamy Sastri.

[6]*Meetings with Remarkable Men.*

[7]*World History of Dance*, p. 245.

[8]*The Dance Through the Ages*, p. 74.

[9]*An Introduction to the Teachings of Bhagwan Shree Rajneesh*, p. 296.

[10]*Eurythmy and the Impulse of Dance*, p. 27.

[11]Lecture given at Interface Foundation, Spring, 1984.

[12]"An Anatomist's Tribute to F. Matthias Alexander," p. 9, from *Man's Supreme Inheritance.*

[13]"An Anatomist's Tribute to F. Matthias Alexander," p. 12.

[14]*Body Awareness in Action*, p. 17.

[15]"The Teaching of F. Matthias Alexander," p. 8.

[16]"An Anatomist's Tribute to F. Matthias Alexander," p. 8.

[17]"An Anatomist's Tribute to F. Matthias Alexander," p. 7.

[18]Frank Jones, notes on the unfinished chapter.

[19]*Body Awareness in Action*, p. 61.

[20]*Body Awareness in Action*, p. 48.

[21]"An Anatomist's Tribute to F. Matthias Alexander," p. 8, quoting Dr. Purpura at the conference on "Brain Mechanisms Underlying Speech and Language."

[22]*Body Movement—Coping with the Environment*, p. 111.

[23]*Body Awareness in Action*, p. 144.

[24]*The Way of Life*, p. 53.

[25]"The Teaching of F. Matthias Alexander," p. 12.
[26]*The Way of Life*, p. 101.

Chapter 3

[1]*The Book of Judgment*, p. 160.
[2]*Sugar Blues*, p. 20.
[3]*An Elementary Treatise Upon the Theory and Practice of the Art of Dancing*, p. 25.
[4]*Introduction to the Teachings of Bhagwan Shree Rajneesh*, p. 296.
[5]*Diet for a Small Planet*.
[6]*Gospel According to Thomas*, p. 5.
[7]*Sugar Blues*, p. 80.
[8]*Book of Judgment*, p. 60.
[9]*East West Journal*, December, 1985.
[10]*Astrology, Nutrition and Health*, p. 10.
[11]*Upanishads*.
[12]*The Potent Self*, p. 103.
[13]Adapted from *The Book of Macrobiotics*, p. 31.
[14]*Man the Unknown*, p. 85.
[15]*The Resurrection of the Body*, p. 92.
[16]*Behold Man*, p. 31.

Chapter 4

[1]"An Anatomist's Tribute to F. Matthias Alexander," p. 14.
[2]*Economy in Body Movement* (yin and yang added by author), p. 31.
[3]*Body Movement—Coping with the Environment*, p. 29.

Chapter 5

[1]*Man the Unknown*, p. 85.
[2]*Behold Man*, p. 93.
[3]"An Anatomist's Tribute to F. Matthias Alexander," p. 7.

Bibliography

Alexander, F. Matthias. *The Use of the Self*. Downey, California: Centerline Press, 1986.

Alexander, F. Matthias. *Constructive Conscious Control of the Individual*. Downey, California: Centerline Press, 1985.

Barlow, Marjory. *The Teaching of F. Matthias Alexander*. London, England: The Alexander Institute, 1965.

Bartenieff, Irmgard and Lewis, Dori. *Body Movement—Coping with the Environment*. New York: Science Publishers, Inc., 1980.

Blasis, Carlo. *An Elementary Treatise Upon the Theory and Practice of the Art of Dancing*. Translated by Mary Stewart Evans. New York: Dover Publications, Inc., 1968.

Carrel, Alexis. *Man the Unknown*. London: Hamilton, 1935.

Dart, Raymond A. *An Anatomists Tribute to F. Matthias Alexander*. London: Sheildrake Press, 1970.

Dart. Raymond A. *Voluntary Musculature in the Human Body: the Double-Spiral Arrangement*. Vol. 1, No. 2, Human Potential. 1968.

Davy, Gudrun and Voors, Bons. *Lifeways*. Gloucestershire, England: Hawthorn Press, 1983.

DeMille, Agnes. *The Book of Dance*. New York: Golden Press, 1963.

Doczi, György. *The Power of Limits*. Boston and London: Shambhala, 1981.

Dufty, William. *Sugar Blues*. New York: Warner Books, 1975.

East West Journal, Dec. 1985.

Feldenkrais, Moshe. *The Potent Self*. New York: Harper & Row, 1985.

Gorman, David. *The Body Moveable*. Vols. I, II and III. Ontario: Ampersand Printing Company, 1981.

Gurdjieff. *Meetings with Remarkable Men*. New York: E.P. Dutton, 1969.

Harwood, Raffe Lundgan. *Eurythmy and the Impulse of Dance*. Dornach, Switzerland: Rufold Steiner Press, 1974.

Haskell, Arnold. *Balletomania Then and Now*. New York: Alfred Knopf, 1977.

Heidenry, Carolyn. *Making the Transition to a Macrobiotic Diet*. Brookline, Massachusetts: Aladdin Press, 1984.

Jansky, Robert Carl. *Astrology, Nutrition and Health*. Rockport, Massachusetts: Para Research, Inc., 1977.

Jones, Frank Pierce. *Body Awareness in Action*. New York: Schocken Books, New York, 1976.

Kaptchuk, Ted. *The Web That Has No Weaver*. New York: Congdon and Weed, Inc., 1983.

Kushi, Michio. *How to See Your Health: Book of Oriental Diagnosis*. Tokyo: Japan Publications, Inc., 1980.

Kushi, Michio. *The Macrobiotic Way*. Wayne, New Jersey: Avery Publishing Group, 1985.

Kushi, Michio. *Oriental Astrology*. Boston, Massachusetts: Kushi Institute Publications, 1981.

Kushi, Michio. *The Book of Macrobiotics—the Universal Way of Health and Happiness*. Tokyo: Japan Publications, Inc., 1977.

Kushi, Michio. *The Book of Dō-In: Exercise for Physical and Spiritual Development*. Tokyo: Japan Publications, Inc., 1979.

Laban, Rudolf and Lawrence, F. C. *Effort: Economy in Body Movement*. Boston: Plays, Inc., 1947–74.

Lad, Dr. Vasant. *Ayurveda—the Science of Self-Healing*. Santa Fe: Lotus Press, 1984.

Lao Tzu. *The Way of Life*. Translation of *Tao Te Ching* by R. B. Blakney. New York: Mentor, 1955.

Lappe, Frances Moor. *Diet for a Small Planet*. New York: Ballantine Books, 1971.

Life, the Editors of. *The Earth* (Life Nature Library). New York: Time, Inc., 1962.

Lutyens, Mary. *Krishnamurti: the Years of Fulfillment*. New York: Ferrar, Straus and Giroux, 1983.

Maisel, Edward (Ed.). *The Resurrection of the Body: The Essential Writings of F.M. Alexander*. New York: Dell Publishing Company, 1974.

Nilsson, Lennart. *Behold Man*. Boston and Toronto: Little, Brown and Company, 1974.

Ohsawa, George. *The Book of Judgment*. Los Angeles: Ignoramus Press, 1966.

Poncé, Charles. *Kabbalah*. Wheaton, Ill.: Quest Books, 1983.

Rajneesh, Bhagwan Shree. *The Book—An Introduction to the Teachings of Bhagwan Shree Rajneesh*. Oregon: Rajneesh International, 1984.

Rudhyar, Dane. *Astrology of Personality*.

Sachs, Curt. *World History of the Dance*. New York: W.W. Norton & Company, Inc., 1963.

Sorell, Walter. *The Dance Through the Ages*. New York: Grosset and Dunlap, 1967.

Thomas. *The Gospel According to Thomas*. New York: Harper and Row, 1959.

Young, Lailan. *Secrets of the Face*. Boston and Toronto: Little, Brown and Company, 1984.

Additional Suggested Reading by These Authors:

Macrobiotics: Aveline Kushi; Wendy and Edward Esko; Shizuko Yamamoto, Ann Marie Colbin, Mary Estella, Dr. Anthony Sattilaro, Alex Jack (information available through the East West Foundation, 17 Station Street, Brookline, MA 02146).

The Alexander Technique: Dr. Wilfred Barlow; Michael Gelb. Books available through Centerline Press, Downey, California.

Index